How Population Change Will Transform Our World

HOW POPULATION CHANGE WILL TRANSFORM OUR WORLD

SARAH HARPER

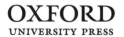

OXFORD
UNIVERSITY PRESS

OXFORD
UNIVERSITY PRESS

Great Clarendon Street, Oxford, OX2 6DP,
United Kingdom

Oxford University Press is a department of the University of Oxford.
It furthers the University's objective of excellence in research, scholarship,
and education by publishing worldwide. Oxford is a registered trade mark of
Oxford University Press in the UK and in certain other countries

First edition published in 2016

Impression: 2

Published in the United States of America by Oxford University Press
198 Madison Avenue, New York, NY 10016, United States of America

British Library Cataloguing in Publication Data
Data available

Library of Congress Control Number: 2015959820

ISBN 978–0–19–878409–8

Printed in Great Britain by
Clays Ltd, St Ives plc

For Imogen

FOREWORD

What Is Myth and What Is Science?

The public mythology surrounding the world's population is clear—the world's population is growing exponentially and out of control, and the reason is that too many women are bearing too many children. Or so it would seem from the media outpourings around migration, population, and family planning. The reality is very different. It is true that some 30 years ago the main population question was 'How can we stop the world population reaching 24 billion by the end of the twenty-first century?' But something which demographers failed to predict was how quickly child-bearing across the world (with the exception of sub-Saharan Africa) would fall. So that now around two-thirds of the world's countries are below, at, or near replacement levels of around two children per couple. As a result, maximum population has now been revised downwards and downwards so that 10 billion is the more likely UN prediction for this century.

A second demographic process which we also failed to see coming was that death rates would fall not only across the life course up until old age, but that they would continue to fall after 65, so that in advanced economies older people would experience longer and longer lives post-retirement, a trend that we are now also seeing in middle income countries as well. As a result of these two process—falling child bearing and falling death rates—the population of the world is slowly ageing, transitioning as it develops economically from countries with very high percentages of children and adolescents, to an increasing number of countries with a booming labour force, to a growing number of a countries with over half their populations aged over 50.

The Oxford Martin School asked if I would write a book which explored this global age shift, drawing on some 20 years of population research by the Oxford Institute of Population Ageing, to highlight the challenges and opportunities such age-structural change was bringing to different regions of the world. It is an opportunity to explode the myths that surround the word 'population'— and to outline the very different picture which the science of demography is bringing to our understanding of twenty-first-century population challenges.

Sarah Harper
University of Oxford

ACKNOWLEDGEMENTS

I wish to thank the Oxford Martin School for encouraging me to write this book. I am particularly grateful for the constant encouragement of the School's founder, James Martin, and his wife Lillian, to explore the ideas presented here. Intellectual stimulation was also provided by conversations with David Bloom, Ron Lee, Michael Hurd, Linda Waite, Francois Farah, Peter Poit, Ron Lesthaeghe, George Leeson, Kenneth Howse, and Tommy Bengtsson, and the valuable words of wisdom of Richard Suzman, who stood by me and supported my research for 20 valuable years.

Latha Menon and Jenny Nugee provided constructive editorial guidance for OUP. This book would not have been completed without the indispensable research and editorial assistance of Nana Nanitashvilli, whom I cannot thank enough.

Finally, my constant gratitude to my long-suffering mother and father, and to George, Imogen, Giles, and Caroline for enduring long discussions on the importance of twenty-first-century demographic change whilst walking, cooking, and running with me as I develop my ideas.

CONTENTS

CONTENTS

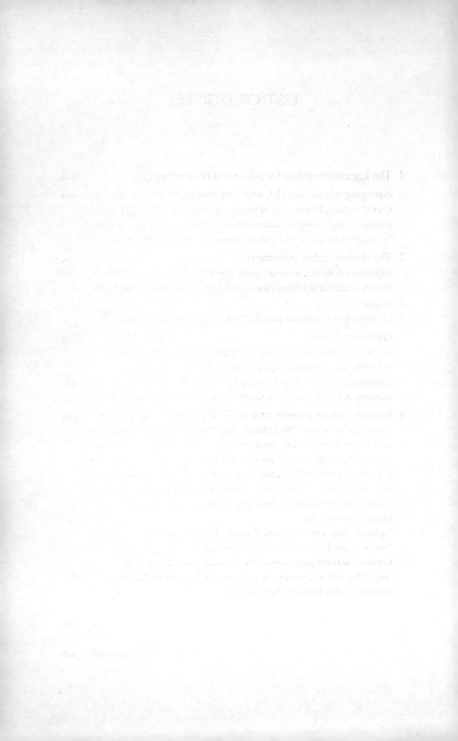

LIST OF FIGURES

The publisher and author apologize for any errors or omissions in
the above list. If contacted they will be pleased to rectify these at
the earliest opportunity.

LIST OF TABLES

CHAPTER ONE

The Age Narrative

The changing age composition of the world

The world is undergoing an unprecedented change in its age composition. This started in Europe in the mid-eighteenth century and took over 200 years to complete. It began in Asia and Latin America during the twentieth century and will be completed in less than 100 years, and is now beginning in Africa. It is the demographic transition, the process by which death rates start to fall, followed by childbearing rates. Why the demographic transition occurred when it did, where it did, and how it did is strongly debated. However, the general pattern is that as humans develop economically, mortality falls, and sometime later fertility falls. It has long been recognized that in the time gap between the two trends population grows rapidly; what is often less understood is the significant change in a country's age composition which occurs as a result.

In terms of the demographic transition and resultant age-structural change, the world can be divided very broadly into three demographic regimes: *advanced economies* moving towards a low percentage of young people and a growing percentage of older people; *emerging economies* dominated by a large percentage of young and mid-life adults sitting between two smaller dependent groups—children and older people; and the *least developed economies* with a very large percentage of children, adolescents, and young people (see Figure 1).[1]

Europe, for example, reached maturity at the turn of the millennium, by the measure of more people over 60 than under 15. Asia will hold a large group of working age until the middle of the century. Then its proportion of young people will start to fall, and in Asia there will be more than 1 billion people over 60, 25 per cent of the population, compared to less than 1 billion under 15, 18 per cent of the population.[2] Similarly, Latin America and the Caribbean will reach 21 per cent age 60 and over by 2040, while those under 15 will fall to 19 per cent. Indeed, by 2050 for the first time there will be the same number of old as young in the world—with 2 billion of each—each accounting for 21 per cent of the world's population. Africa, however, will continue to grow and remain young. It is projected to more than double in size by 2050 from 1 to 2.5 billion, with 32.2 per cent of its population still under 15 by the middle of the century.[3] As a result, the global distribution of people will also change, with an overall increase in those living in Asia and Africa, and a fall in European and North American populations. The emerging economies, predominantly in Asia and Latin America, and the least developed countries, mainly in sub-Saharan Africa, will account for 97 per cent of the growth leading up to 2050. Asia will comprise 54 per cent of the world population by 2050 at 5 billion, while Europe will decline from 738 to 708 million, only around 7 per cent of the global population.

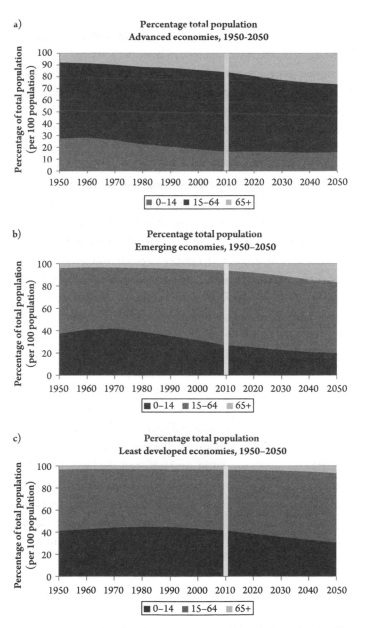

a)

**Percentage total population
Advanced economies, 1950-2050**

b)

**Percentage total population
Emerging economies, 1950–2050**

c)

**Percentage total population
Least developed economies, 1950–2050**

FIG 1 The age composition for advanced economies (a), emerging economies (b), and least developed economies (c)

The demographic drivers of change

The classic demographic transition is typically associated with economic development, and is perceived as comprising four main stages[4] (Figure 2). In stage 1, populations experience high death rates from disease, famine, malnutrition, and lack of clean water and sanitation; there is no impetus, or even the thought to reduce fertility. These populations have high birth and death rates, and a relatively small but often fluctuating population size—for example England pre-1780, and current-day Ethiopia. Stage 2 sees improvements in public heath, sanitation, clean water, and food, and mortality, especially infant and child mortality, falls. There are, however, still high fertility rates, resulting in a rapidly expanding population size—for example nineteenth-century England and current-day Sudan. In stage 3 rapidly falling total fertility rates[5] occur alongside low mortality rates. There is a still expanding but slowing population size such as

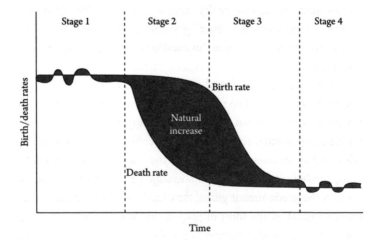

FIG 2 The demographic transition

England in the early twentieth century and twenty-first century Uruguay. Stage 4 sees low mortality and fertility, a high but relatively stable population—current-day UK and Canada, for example.[6]

Most countries of the developed world are now in the late stages of the demographic transition, resulting in the decrease in both mortality and fertility rates, which typically is associated with economic development. Mortality rates fall first, including infant mortality, enabling the survival of large birth cohorts into adulthood. Falls in fertility occur with economic development, which leads to family planning, education, and employment opportunities for women. They also appear directly linked to a response to falling infant mortality rates themselves. Population growth levels off and the profile of the population ages as late-life death rates fall and individuals survive to increasingly older ages. The steady increase in life expectancy is thus occurring in the context of population ageing, whereby falling fertility rates have led to increasing percentages of older dependents, and falling percentages of economically active workers. The fact that increasing longevity is occurring within populations which are themselves ageing has clear implications for providing for this longevity.

A third demographic trend, migration, has a potentially strong and long-lasting impact on population growth and structure through the interaction between the number of migrants, their relatively young age structure, and their higher fertility. For example, many advanced economies have relied on the migration of workers to compensate for their own population ageing. For more than half a century the predominant global flow has been the immigration of human capital, in the form of migrant workers, from poor young countries in the South (southern hemisphere—Asia, Africa, and Latin America) to the rich old countries of the North—(predominantly the US and the European former colonial powers, such as Great Britain, France, and the Iberian countries of Spain and Portugal), in exchange for economic capital—provided both from national governments and multinational corporations, and in the form of individual remittances. Similarly, some emerging economies, which have a burgeoning cohort of young people, are exporting their workers to other countries where the labour markets are more buoyant. This may be via direct support of outmigration, such as the arrangements of the government of the Philippines to send women to work overseas in the health and care sectors of richer nations, or the facilitation by some Indian states, such as Kerala, to enable young Indian men to work in the oil-rich Middle East. In both cases, the sending countries benefit from the large flow of remittances sent back by the workers, and the host countries gain much needed labour in certain sectors of their economies. However, while these are important movements, and will be discussed later in the book, they cannot compensate for the overall age-structural change propelled by the significant momentum of fertility and mortality decline.

Three lives...

The stories of three women born in 1975

SAMIRA, NIGER

Shortly after her thirteenth birthday, Samira's parents married her, their eldest daughter, to a 52-year-old friend of her father. Her first child, a girl, was born one year later, and now at 40 Samira has experienced some 15 pregnancies, and has given birth to nine live babies. All of her four daughters were married by 13. Samira became a grand-mother at 27, was widowed at 28, and now has 24 grandchildren.

Samira sees herself as fortunate. Unlike several of her friends, who were also married to much older men at a very young age, she escaped the damage and death caused by very young childbirth, and all but one of her children are still alive. Her eldest daughter was not so lucky. She died in childbirth at 12. Young girls are particularly vulnerable to complications in labour, and childbirth can result in an obstetric fistula (a hole in the birth canal), which leaves women permanently incontinent and sometimes ostracized from their communities. Samira has a limited education, like 98 per cent of Niger girls she left school before secondary education, and like half of the girls in her village she was married by the age of 13. Samira rarely leaves the village where she lives; she has been completely dependent on her husband's family to provide her and her children with housing, food, and clothing. She is also preparing her eldest granddaughter for marriage within the year, arranged for the 11 year old by her future husband's family. Samira can expect to become a great-grandmother in her early 40s and live into her 60s, and will see many great-grandchildren born before she dies, and maybe even her great-great-grandchildren.

Niger, Samira's home, is a country with the highest childbearing rate in the world, each woman on average bearing seven children.[7] It also has one of the highest mortality rates, with infant mortality at 60 per 1,000 live births, maternal mortality at 690 per 100,000 live births, and a life expectancy at birth of only 61 years. Niger has one of the lowest educational rates in the world, with only 5 per cent enrolment in secondary school, less than 2 per cent of girls. Over one-quarter of girls are married by 15, rising to 60 per cent by age 19, and far higher in rural communities, where the majority are married at 12 or 13. As life expectancy is slowly rising, but early first birth continues, the possibility of many generations being alive at the same time is increasing.

Varya left her home in a small town in southern Malaysia when she was 16, having dropped out of secondary education early, and travelled to Singapore. Here she found a job as a cleaner in a large American-owned hotel. Her early years in the city were difficult, and she spent ten years living in a hostel and undertaking menial work. At 28, on a return visit to see her family, she agreed to marry a local boy of her age. They had been at primary school together and he now worked in a local factory in the town. Varya was insistent that she kept her job at the hotel, as she was now working in housekeeping, had learned good English, and was happy with her work, which she saw as well paid. After her marriage, she travelled daily by bus across the border from Malaysia to Singapore, a two-hour journey each way, undertaking 12-hour shifts, six days a week. Eventually, at age 33, she agreed under pressure from her husband to have a child. The hotel was very accommodating, and six months after the birth of her son Varya was back working and commuting, her son being cared for full-time by her husband's mother. Varya continues to work in the Singapore hotel, now as a restaurant waitress. Her husband's job has also improved, and he now works for a new international firm which has relocated to Malaysia, travelling to work in the US on three separate occasions. Despite the good money they are both now earning, Varya and her husband have decided to stop at one child. They wish for their son to have the 'best of everything'—the possessions and opportunities which they were denied.

Malaysia, Varya's birth country, has changed considerably during her lifetime. Varya's mother left school at 12, at a time when only 19 per cent of girls had a secondary education. Varya's mother bore eight babies, six of whom survived to adulthood, and she died when Varya was a child. Now Malaysia has a high rate of female education: 66 per cent enrolment in secondary school with 82 per cent completion at 16. The average age at marriage is 25.7 and at first birth has reached 30.5. The delaying of first births and spacing of any subsequent births has reduced Malaysia's childbearing rate to just over two. Neighbouring Singapore has one of the lowest childbearing rates in the world, at just over one. Varya intends to work in Singapore for another 15 years, and then retire. She can expect to live into her 70s,[8] and if she becomes a grandmother, it may be just before she dies.

LISA, ITALY

Following her degree in Milan, Lisa moved to Rome and then to London to work in publishing. She enjoyed the international community within which she worked and lived, made new friends easily, and had several relationships. She regularly travelled back to the small town in northern Italy where she was born and grew up, to see her parents and her younger brother, who still remained living at home. At 37, she met her current partner, a Chilean man working in PR. They have lived together for the past three years, and consider London to be their home. Lisa worries about her parents: though currently still young in their 60s she is concerned about their old age when she is not around to help and support them. She also knows that her mother is disappointed that neither she nor her brother have had children. Of the 20 girls in Lisa's school class, less than half have borne their first child; Lisa does think about having a family, but worries that they will not be able to afford their lifestyle with a child; she is also concerned not to disrupt her very successful publishing career which she really enjoys. Given current pension changes in the UK, Lisa expects to continue working until she is 70, and still enjoy 10 to 15 years of active retirement. When she retires, her parents may well still be alive, and she feels that this would be a good time to return to Italy, to look after them.

Italy, Lisa's birth home, has one of the lowest childbearing rates in the world,[9] and 57.6 per cent of women go on to tertiary education. Age at first marriage is 30.1 and maternal age at first birth is very high, at 31.06 years, with 22 per cent of women age 40 still childless. Life expectancy is high, with both men and women expecting to live well into their 80s. If Lisa does have a baby, the child can expect to live to over 100.

These three vignettes[10] illustrate the contrasting life chances of women alive in the second decade of the twenty-first century, lives framed by the interaction of changes across an individual's life course with the changing societal context within which these lives are experienced. Numerous factors will influence these lives— economic, social, political, etc.—including the demography of the time. Demographic factors will shape whether these lives are long and healthy, or short and threatened by disease and ill health; they will frame whether the individual grows up in a large birth cohort attracting a large percentage of resources from other generations, or needing to compete with others of the same generation for limited societal assets, including employment, housing, and marriage partners; and they will affect whether an individual has many or few siblings, and whether they live in multigenerational families. While in many countries individuals can choose whether to marry early or late, and bear many or few children themselves, these decisions are also influenced by the prevailing norms of the time, and in some places these choices are not choices at all for the individual.

... in three regions

Advanced economies here comprise the UN more developed regions (see Appendix 1). These are predominantly European and North American, and also include Australia and New Zealand. Many are also OECD (Organisation for Economic Co-operation and Development) countries. In addition, demographically Japan fits more closely with the advanced economies than with emerging economies. Advanced economies are affected by three dominant demographic trends: a fertility rate below replacement level; unprecedented and continuing declines in late-life mortality; and relatively high levels of inward migration (Box 1). The average total fertility rate (TFR) is 1.67, life expectancy at birth is 78.3 and at 60 is 22.8. This is resulting in societies with a decline in the proportion of younger people, both child dependents and those of working and reproducing age; an increase in the proportion and number of older people, in particular the oldest old, over age 85; and a more ethnically diverse composition. In addition, 16.4 per cent of their population is under 15, 65.9 per cent of working age, a 17.6 per cent over 65 (Figure 1a).

Most emerging economies lie within Asia, Latin America, and the MENA (Middle East and North Africa) region. Emerging economies are affected by a rapidly falling national total fertility level, which is low among urban and affluent women and still high among rural and poor women; falling mortality rates across the life course leading to increasing life expectancy rates; and high rural to urban migration and national outmigration of skilled workers. There is considerable variation in TFR, both between the countries themselves and within countries, particularly between rural and urban areas. The spectrum of TFR is between 1.7 and 5.7, and life expectancy at birth is 49.2 to 83.7, and at 60 it is 13.7 to 25.8. These societies have a decline in the proportion of child dependents, an increase in the percentage of those of working and reproductive ages, and a small but growing increase in the proportion and number of older people, though often without the institutional structures to support this growing number of elderly dependents.

BOX 1

Advanced economies are affected by:
- a fertility rate below replacement level
- unprecedented and continuing declines in late-life mortality
- relatively high levels of inward migration

Resulting in societies with:
- a decline in the proportion of younger people
- an increase in the proportion and number of older adults
- an increase in the proportion and number of the oldest old
- a more ethnically diverse composition

Emerging economies are affected by:
- a rapidly falling national total fertility level, which is low among urban and affluent women and still high among rural and poor women
- increasing life expectancies, though often without the institutional structures to support the growing number of elderly dependents
- high rural to urban migration and outmigration of skilled workers

Resulting in societies with:
- a decline in the proportion of child dependents
- a high percentage of population of productive age
- a small but growing increase in the proportion and number of older people
- rapid urbanization and need to retain skilled labour

Least developed economies are affected by:
- a high total fertility level, especially among rural and poor women, which is beginning to fall, though also experiencing stalling
- limited reduction in infant and maternal mortality rates
- high rural to urban migration

Resulting in societies with:
- a high proportion of child dependents
- an increasing percentage of population of productive age
- rapid urbanization and need to develop skilled labour

NOTE: Advanced economies, Emerging economies, and Least developed economies are broadly comparable to the High, Medium, and Low Income countries used by economists.

In addition, 25.8 per cent of their population is under 15, 67 per cent of working age, and 6.9 per cent over 65 (Figure 1b). They are also subject to rapid urbanization and need to retain skilled labour.

The least developed economies are defined here as the UN least developed regions. With a few exceptions from Asia, such as Bangladesh, Afghanistan, and Cambodia, they are predominantly located in sub-Saharan Africa. In contrast to the other groupings, the least developed economies are affected by a high total fertility level, especially among rural and poor women, which is beginning to fall, though also experiencing a stalling above replacement level; limited reduction in infant and maternal mortality rates; and high rural to urban migration. The average TFR is 4.27, while life expectancy at birth is still only 62.1 and at 60 is 17.3. These societies still have a high proportion of child dependents and of young adults of working and reproductive age, often without the education and skills required to drive the economy; and they are experiencing rapid urbanization. Forty per cent of their population is under 15, 56.5 per cent of working age, and 3.6 per cent over 65 (Figure 1c).

The impact of age-structural change

The debate in all three demographic zones needs to be framed though an understanding of the interaction of changes at the individual and at the societal level, bearing in mind that these will also be mediated by the increasingly global interconnectedness of the world. Most of Asia and Latin America are currently experiencing a rapid growth in workers, which are now growing faster than any other group. Africa still has high growth rates in children, but will soon experience a rapid expansion in its population of working age. Europe and North America are past this stage and are facing fewer workers and children, and a growth in older adults. China and some South East Asian countries will be in this position very shortly. In light of these significantly changing age structures, the challenge in all regions is how to sustain and enhance well-being across an individual's life, while at the same time reducing the inequalities within each generation, and ensuring an equitable reallocation of resources between the generations. As countries develop, so their citizens are able to access the benefits of social, economic, and scientific advances. In all societies, however, some people are better able to access these resources than others. How these resources are distributed accounts for the inequalities within societies. Demographically there are two main types of inequality: that within a generation—intragenerational inequality—which is mainly mediated by socio-economic, ethnic, and gender factors; and that between generations—intergenerational inequalities— or between different birth cohorts. In particular, it may be argued that large generations take more societal resources than smaller ones. This may be mediated by market forces: for example rapid growth in the numbers entering the labour market may depress wage levels for all, or an increase in the number of older people, who are likely to have assets, may reduce overall interest rates. Or they may influence government policies: in advanced economies there is a current need to transfer societal resources towards the large cohorts of older adults; in emerging economies, the desire by governments to utilize the large cohorts of working age to drive the economy can threaten to reduce the societal resources available to the dependent generations on either side—children and old people; while in the least developed world, emphasis is often placed by governments on the very young, as they are the future of the country. However, this reallocation of resources to ensure intergenerational equity is also often overshadowed by the huge inequalities within each generation—between those able to access resources in health, education, and income, and those less able to.

Advanced economies

In advanced economies, not only are individuals living longer, they are doing so within a population which is in itself growing older. To grow old in a society where most people are young is fundamentally different from doing so in a society where most people are old. In demographically young populations, there are high proportions of economically active individuals who may produce the wealth needed to support dependents, old and young. However, these societies may not place much emphasis on the well-being of older people, as they comprise a small minority of the overall population. Conversely, demographically old populations have a lower proportion of economically active individuals, and thus the responsibility of providing for old age dependency may increasingly fall to the older person themselves. A key question for these societies is not only maintaining well-being across the life course of these longer lived individuals, but also how we redistribute resources within this new demographic.

The argument here is that all humans currently experience a decline in mental and physical capacity as they age. This can be mediated by lifestyle/environment, and increasingly in the future by biomedical intervention, which may delay, though probably not prevent, the onset of this decline. This decline leads to an increased individual need for health and social care, and for a source of late-life income, usually in the form of a pension. There are, however, significant inequalities in the process of this decline, which is reflected both in the concepts of life expectancy (how long groups of people live on average) and healthy life expectancy (how long they may live without disability). Such inequalities are closely related to socio-economic, gender, and ethnic difference. Given that some decline is inevitable, societies also need to ensure that those who are experiencing this decline are also able to maintain a high level of well-being. The ability of an individual to maintain well-being is compromised first by actual increases in dependency as their mental and physical abilities decline, and second by society constructing dependency, through such policies as requiring early withdrawal—retirement—from economic activity on grounds of age while the individual is actually still healthy and productive. Furthermore, in trying to maintain population well-being, societies which have a growing proportion of their populations in old age have to consider how to redistribute resources within this new demographic. In other words, to move resources away from a focus on younger people towards older people in an equitable manner, both intergenerationally (between the generations) and intragenerationally (within each generation).

These factors—increasing decline and dependency, inequality, and equitable redistribution of resources—frame the major challenges for advanced economies.

Emerging economies

Individuals within emerging economies are experiencing a reduction in mortality across their lives. The chances of themselves, their children, and their grandchildren dying as babies, youths, and young adults have been significantly reduced. They and their parents can expect an extension of life expectancy at older ages, and thus live well into old age. In addition, the childbearing rate of women has fallen, especially in urban areas. This is due to women delaying having their first child, increasing the spaces between each child, and bearing fewer babies in total. As a consequence men and women in the labour market have fewer children to look after, and can focus more of their resources on economic activity. The delaying of first childbirth enables women to increase the time they spend in education as well as in the labour market. Indeed, it may be argued that retaining girls in school longer is an important factor behind the delaying of first births. The lower rates of childbearing have a particular importance in enabling women to undertake paid employment. Again, there are significant inequalities in this experience, with still high levels of childbearing, morbidity or ill health, and mortality in the less developed rural areas.

At the population level, many of these societies have experienced a sudden fall in childbearing after a time of high numbers of births. This, combined with a fall in mortality rates for younger men and women, especially maternal mortality rates, means that a large proportion of their population is now of productive age, and in particular many of these societies have a *youth bulge* of young adults under 25. A key challenge for these societies is ensuring that education, health, and governance structures are sufficiently and appropriately established to provide labour markets which may produce jobs for the growing number of these young adults. If successful, this may result in a *demographic dividend*.[11] At the same time, these societies need to ensure that elementary education is available for all and that health provision is maintained, especially for children, women, and the growing number of older people who are surviving to older ages. They must also tackle the growing inequalities between the burgeoning, typically urban middle classes and the rural poor, and inequalities within urban areas themselves, including providing infrastructure for sprawling urban growth. In addition, there is a need to redistribute resources to the urban and rural poor while still maintaining the much needed economic growth to support raising standards of living for all.

These factors—increasing unemployment and youth disengagement, inequality, and the equitable redistribution of resources alongside promoting economic growth—frame the major challenges for emerging economies.

Least developed economies

Individuals within the least developed countries, the majority of which are in sub-Saharan Africa, are still experiencing relatively high levels of childbearing, and of disease and death across the life course. Women are still likely to undergo continual pregnancy, and experience miscarriages, stillbirths, and the deaths of their infants, as well as expect their children to die before adulthood. They themselves, their sisters, adult daughters, and even their own mothers face injury or death from childbearing and childbirth. While there is a decline in infant and maternal mortality across the region and in a growing number of countries, the possibility of choosing the number of children to bear, limited family planning programmes, poor health conditions, and gender inequality are slowing down the decline in both childbearing and infant and child deaths. Continued high fertility rates supporting rapid population growth are still threatening the well-being of individuals in these poorest countries. Even where fertility is declining, given the very young age structure of these countries, and the large number of women of reproductive age living there, high numbers of children will still be born for many decades to come—the so-called *demographic momentum* effect. The shift in the age structure from high child dependency to a population of predominantly working age is a long way away for most of the least developed countries, and the large size of the young population in relation to the working-age population will delay any demographic dividend for several decades.

In addition, alongside disease and high birth rates, many countries are still grappling with extreme poverty, famine, and civil conflict, and have barely been able to develop advanced systems of education, health, and governance. Educational opportunities for girls, particularly at the secondary level, remain limited, and most of the working population is underskilled. Inadequate governance, limited regulation, and weak institutions lead to high levels of corruption and low respect for legal systems, property rights, and contracts. Physical infrastructure remains inefficient in many countries with poor communication systems, including roads, railways, and telecommunications, and unreliable water and sanitation, food production, and distribution.

These factors—high fertility, rapid population growth, high levels of disease and mortality, poor health, education, and governance systems, a continuing very young dependent population, and a low-skilled working population—frame the major challenges for the least developed countries.

Economic and societal consequences

The decline in the proportion of younger people in a population is seen to lead to a decline in economic activity and an increase in the proportion of older people, with the resulting economic burdens of increased requirement for pensions and health care. These predictions arise from the notion that generally productive capacity varies across the life course, flowing from a period of youth dependency, through high productive potential in adulthood, and returning to a decrease in productive capacity in old age. When we are young adults we produce, consume, and save, and when we are older we reduce our production and consumption and begin to draw down on our investments. This concern is amplified as increases in longevity lead to older people receiving publically funded pensions for a greater length of time. In addition, it is assumed that older populations have lower rates of consumption and will draw down on savings accumulated in both private and national accounts. Even if older people increase their working years, thus delaying the uptake of their pensions, there is also the presumption that older labour forces are less innovative and have lower productivity than younger ones.

The macroeconomic effects will differ depending upon the age composition of the population. Large birth cohorts, especially if sandwiched on each side by smaller ones, have a measureable economic impact. As babies grow into children, so resources must be diverted from other areas to provide housing, schooling, medical care, etc. Such a diversion of resources may lead to a slowdown in economic growth. As the children grow into young adults, their labour, if supported by the right institutional structures, may lead to enhanced economic growth. And as a large cohort begins to age, so there may be a decline in productivity again as they cease economic activity, draw down on pensions, and require extra resources to provide sufficient old-age health and social care.

One way to explore the impacts of this age-structural change is to consider how consumption versus production alters a society's age. In all societies, dependent children and dependent older adults consume more resources than they produce, while those of working age, however defined, produce more than they consume. This does not negate the input of older adults to non-economic activities such as caring, advice, and support, which comprises an essential role within most societies, and allows those of working age to be more productive. Economists have tried to measure these impacts through an analysis of how each group within a society produces, consumes, saves, and shares resources. They argue that the economic lifecycle works through the flow of resources over time across generations, mediated by a complex of social, political, and economic institutions.[12]

Figure 3 neatly illustrates this relationship for two countries at different stages of the demographic transition and thus with

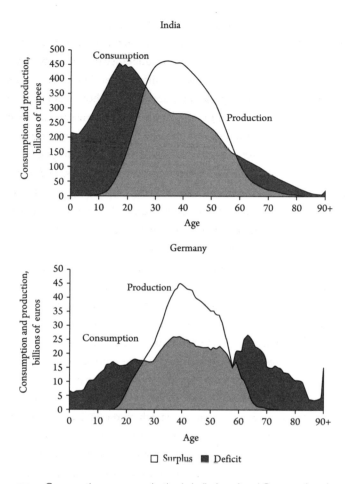

India

Germany

□ Surplus ■ Deficit

FIG 3 Consumption versus production in India (2004) and Germany (2003)

very different age structures. In both countries, consumption exceeds production for long periods of life, with high consumption over production among the young in India, and among the old in Germany.

The support ratio—number of workers to number of consumers—is a useful measure of the changing relationship between producers and consumers. Those countries at the beginning of the age-structural shift will have a low number of workers to consumers—a low support ratio—as there are so many children. Africa, for example, has a low number of producers to consumers—66 per 100—due to its high childbearing rate and large proportion of child dependents, but this figure is forecast to rise to 86 per 100 by the middle of the century. By contrast East Asia, with its current high levels of workers, but low dependents, will fall from 90 producers per 100 consumers currently to only 70 producers per 100. And Europe, already well along the age transition, will fall from 84 producers per 100 currently to reach 69 by 2050, with some European countries as low as 50 due to the growing percentage of older dependents.

In some emerging economies, such as Indonesia, the Philippines, and Thailand, increased taxes from the growing proportion of workers will offset the benefits needed as their populations age; but in most other countries tax revenue will fall as the countries start to age. However, it is also argued that as fertility falls, so investment in children via increased health and education raises the 'human capital' of the future working population. This to an extent offsets the decline in the numbers of workers, as each becomes more productive.

Economists typically believe that the demographic transition is something which follows on from economic growth; demographers believe that it is a more complex process driven by socio-cultural as well as economic factors. Indeed, some go as far as to suggest that the demographic transition's implications for the economy are greater than economic factors for the transition, and that the transition has played as important a role in the process of human development. Figure 4 demonstrates these combined forces by

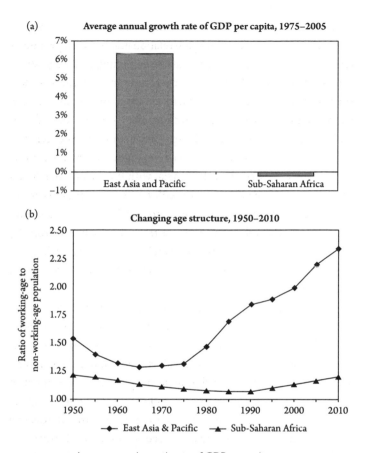

(a) **Average annual growth rate of GDP per capita, 1975–2005**

East Asia and Pacific   Sub-Saharan Africa

(b) **Changing age structure, 1950–2010**

Ratio of working-age to non-working-age population

1950 1960 1970 1980 1990 2000 2010

East Asia & Pacific   Sub-Saharan Africa

FIG 4 Average annual growth rate of GDP per capita, 1975–2005

comparing East Asia and sub-Saharan Africa, two economically and demographically extreme regions. Here we can see the extraordinary growth experienced in East Asia during the late twentieth century, with an annual average rate of growth of GDP of some 6.4 per cent. This has been termed the 'East Asian miracle'. During the same period, sub-Saharan Africa experienced zero growth, with annual average GDP actually falling by 0.2 per cent. However, when considering the age-structural change in East Asia across this time, we can see the impact of a large working-age population (defined as the population aged 15–64) relative to the non-working-age population—both children and old-age 'dependents' (defined as the population under age 15 and over age 65, respectively). As is clear, the ratio of working-age people to dependents was lower in sub-Saharan Africa than in East Asia throughout the entire period. While East Asia had higher numbers of people working and saving, sub-Saharan Africa had a high burden of youth dependency, due to its long history of high fertility. East Asia has more than 2.3 workers for every non-worker, sub-Saharan Africa has 1.2 workers per non-worker, which may be described as every Asian household having an entire extra worker for every non-worker.[13]

Inequalities

Many governments are not only concerned with economic growth, they also wish to reduce inequalities. Inequalities may be defined in economic terms as unequal access to income or assets,[14] or in a wider definition as unequal access to wider resources such as educational opportunities, health, and environmental resources. Some wish to reduce inequality in order to promote economic performance, others may wish to address social problems, still others may wish for a fairer society as the end in itself.[15] It is regarded by many as a moral good that a civilized society strives to ensure that all its citizens have equal access to that society's resources. This is certainly a view this book takes.

Economists and others debate as to whether unequal societies, in terms of income and other assets, lead to poorer economic outcomes for both the individual and the country, which impacts upon growth. The evidence seems inconclusive. However, in terms of other measures, such as health, many argue that populations tend to have overall poorer health outcomes if there are higher levels of inequality.

Most research in this area has explored income inequality within a country in terms of the existing population at the time. We can have differences within a single generation or, to be more technically correct, a single birth cohort: i.e. those people who were born within a single year or more commonly with a group of years, say a decade. The socio-economic circumstances into which we are born help to shape our life chances—our educational opportunities, health circumstances, income, and wealth trajectory. Our sex and ethnicity also have an influence. There are also differences between birth cohorts. The time we are born into may give us access to certain resources or exclude us from other opportunities—the UK cohort born in the post-war period had access to free National Health Service care from birth, which improved health outcomes in relation to previous cohorts; the millennium cohort has had access to the Internet since it was born, which will shape many of their life opportunities.

The recognition that a change in the age structure of a country may be an important driver has been more recently recognised.[16] There has been particular interest in the way these changes alter the size of different demographic groups which then alter the distribution of income, particularly at the household level. Of particular interest is the role of different sized birth cohorts. It has long been argued, for example, that when a large birth cohort enters the labour market its entry wage falls, and this fall may persist across their working lives with associated effects on delayed marriage and childbearing.[17] In addition, when these large cohorts age, social policies may be enacted to increase old-age benefits so the smaller cohorts coming up behind may face increased taxes or social security contributions to pay for these. Such factors lead to inequalities in income between different birth cohorts.[18] Furthermore, resources flow from one generation to another. Within households these may be from parents to dependent children, or from adult children to dependent parents; public transfers occur via a taxation system, whereby taxes and other working-age payments flow, for example, via the provision of schools and pensions to support younger and older dependents respectively.

Another key factor is the change in household structure, which some argue is a more important driver of changing inequality than cohort factors. Smaller households, especially single households, tend to be worse off than large ones, where there are economies of scale. Demographic drivers are important here. Falling fertility increases the proportion of young single and couple households and the length of time young people stay in this household type; falling mortality increases the proportion of elderly couples and single occupied households, and again the length of time individuals remain thus.[19]

The challenge

As the twentieth century was drawing to a close, the overwhelming population question was how could world population be prevented from growing to over 20 billion during the next century. Yet, within a couple of decades, demographic predictions had shifted from rampant growth to declining and ageing populations. Now the defining demographic characteristics of the twenty-first century are likely to be declining births and stabilization in size, and maximum world population is predicted to increase from the current 7 billion to around 11 billion by the end of the current century.[20] Presently, in many countries the working-age population outnumbers the combined population of old and young; globally there are five times the number of those of working age than those over 60 for example. However, by 2050 this will almost have halved to just 2.9. Not only will the large working-age cohorts start to enter older age, in many countries they will also benefit from the lengthening of lives, so many will survive for far longer, living into their 80s and even 90s.

The challenge therefore is to maintain well-being across the life course, including extending healthy life expectancy, reducing inequalities within generations, and at the same time ensuring equity between generations as societal resources are reallocated to the larger generations. The question is, how will different countries at varying stages of the age transition cope with this challenge?

CHAPTER TWO

How Did We Get Here?

The drivers of change

It is early in the nineteenth century and two small rivers run through the small town of Witham in the English county of Essex. Along each river huddle crowded small cottages, occupied by adults and children, pigs, chickens, and goats, and a number of open slaughter houses, the refuse and manure from both spilling out into the lanes and streams. In between lie open sewers moving large amounts of foul-smelling effluent which flows directly into the rivers. Children play among the piles of human and animal manure, collected by the townsmen and women to dry and sell. It is a town of cholera, typhus, and tuberculosis, a town no different from many in the country at the time. Indeed, disease caused by such conditions was the biggest cause of death among the English population.[1] Over 80 per cent of all the deaths in the late eighteenth and early nineteenth century were caused by diseases such as cholera, typhus, typhoid, and even malaria, far exceeding death from old age. Death across the life course at all ages was commonplace, and half the population died before they reached their mid-40s. Yet Europe was already in the grasp of one of the biggest demographic changes known to mankind—the great *European transition*. Mortality rates were slowly but steadily declining. While there were still crises such as epidemics and famine, there was a steady overall decline in the death rate. Within a few decades, fertility rates would mirror these falls.

Sanitation and clean water

Public health initiatives played a large role in the decline of European mortality throughout the nineteenth century. England in the 1830s and 1840s witnessed two influenza epidemics and the appearance of cholera. Asiatic cholera arrived in Sunderland during the autumn of 1831. A waterborne disease, it rapidly travelled both north to Scotland and south to London, claiming over 50,000 lives. Barely had this first epidemic died out when it returned, accompanied this time by other epidemics of influenza, typhus, and typhoid which ravaged the country from 1836 to 1842. Cholera is usually picked up through contaminated water or food. The rapid dehydration caused by extreme diarrhoea can kill within hours. In the crowded unsanitary conditions of the early nineteenth century, when most waste was disposed of in open sewers or in the streets, flowing into the rivers that provided drinking water, the spread of cholera was almost uncontrollable. From the late eighteenth century onwards in London, for example, the affluent property-owning classes had begun to install water-flushing closets which distributed their own effluent into the local rivers and other waterways from which the population obtained their drinking water.[2]

It was not just England which was thus afflicted; cities, towns, and villages throughout Europe were the same. The nineteenth-century Italian city of Florence has been described as akin to a six-teenth-century city with poor hygiene and overcrowding,[3] creating an ideal environment for the epidemics which ravaged the city: Typhus in 1801 and 1818, followed by four consecutive outbreaks of cholera between 1835 and 1867, and a steady growth in deaths from tuberculosis.[4] Poor sanitation and overcrowding in Paris contributed to the spread of cholera there in 1832, with Spain and Portugal being affected in 1833, and by 1837 the epidemic had reached Austria, the German states, the Baltic ports, and Poland, with a mortality rate of 50 per cent.

However, from the middle of the nineteenth century onwards, mortality rates in many parts of Europe began steadily to improve. Importantly, the relationship of these epidemics to the unsanitary conditions in which the population lived became increasingly recognized.[5] Between 1750 and 1850, England, France, and Sweden had gained less than one month of life expectancy per year. However, from 1850 to 1900, this more than doubled to two months per year, driven by improvements in living standards and public health initiatives around sanitation which enabled clean water, improved hygiene, and safe sewage disposal.

Take the city of Florence, for example. In 1865 it became the capital of Italy, and a major restructuring of the old city commenced, with the widespread demolition of crowded housing, the installation of a new sewer system, and fresh water being piped across the city.[6] These improvements in sanitation were followed by a near halving of the death rate in the 100 years between 1790 and 1890.[7] Over the 100 years between 1850 and 1950, two-thirds of the reduction in deaths across the life course in Italy was due to controlling infectious, respiratory, and intestinal diseases. And two-thirds of this reduction in deaths occurred in babies and children under 15. It was a similar story in Germany. In 1892, Max von Pettenkofer, a German pioneer of public health, prevented an outbreak in Munich by starting treatment of the wastewater system. It was the same in London and the other cities and large towns of Britain.[8] The Public Health Acts of 1848 and 1872 established a

General Board of Health and a widespread network of local sanitary authorities which enabled Britain to escape the later European epidemics of cholera.[9]

The role of nutrition

It was not just improved sanitation and clean drinking water which were making a difference. Food availability and production steadily improved across the century. Throughout the eighteenth and nineteenth century, the trade, distribution, and transport systems transformed agriculture from a subsistence to a commercial enterprise, significantly increasing the availability of food.[10] From the eighteenth century, new farming techniques enabled fresh meat to become available all year round, and improved transport allowed fresh fish to reach a greater proportion of the European population. While in the seventeenth and eighteenth centuries meat consumption in Europe was restricted to the privileged few, by the beginning of the nineteenth century the absence of meat in the working man's diet was no longer seen as normal, but increasingly as a form of deprivation.[11] The science of nutrition emerged, with dietary standards being developed in the nineteenth century. Indeed, the 1864 guideline for daily protein consumption of 81 grams of pure protein for a man and 77 grams for a woman are remarkably close to modern recommendations.[12] At the same time, a wider variety of fruit and vegetables were grown, and bottling in 1804 followed by canning in 1820 was successfully developed to preserve these throughout the year.[13] Across the century, European factory food processing was developed. For example, a survey of the Swiss food industry found that chocolate was being produced commercially (1819), and it was followed by pasta (1839), condensed milk and baby foods (1867), powdered soup (1867), margarine (1889) and biscuits (1899).[14]

These commercial initiatives were supported by government-backed public health moves which promoted the safe storage and handling of food. In England and Wales, for example, a variety of Acts laid down by Parliament addressed food hygiene and quality: the 1870s Adulteration of Foods Acts—leading to the appointment of professional inspectors and public analysts by most local authorities in the 1880s; the 1878 and 1889 Weights and Measures Acts; and the 1899 Sale of Food and Drugs Act. The overall result was that throughout the nineteenth century individual nutrition was considerably improved, resulting in a healthier population better able to withstand the ravages of disease.[15]

It should be noted, however, that there were regional and local differences. Historical studies[16] of the Nordic countries, for example, suggest that disease transmission played a bigger part, with the poor farmers in the mountainous regions having lower mortality than their lowland neighbours due to their isolation, particularly in the winter months, from contagious diseases such as smallpox, which ravaged the families of the wealthy, well-nourished, valley populations.

The introduction of pharmaceuticals

While the eighteenth and nineteenth centuries had seen massive reductions in mortality through the improvement in living conditions, the twentieth century saw the steady but increased role of scientific discoveries tackling disease. The large reduction in mortality across the twentieth century was primarily due to the conquering of infections and infectious diseases (Figure 5). The first three decades of the twentieth century saw a significant reduction in deaths,[17] with the introduction of basic but effective pharmaceuticals—Salvarsan in 1910, Sulfonamide drugs in the 1930s, and in particular the discovery of penicillin in 1940 by Sir Alexander

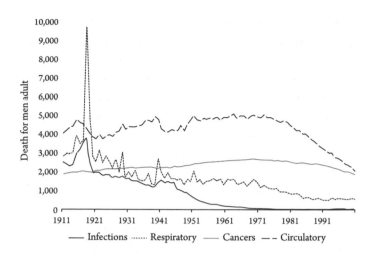

FIG 5 Mortality by major cause: UK, 1911–2005, males

NOTE: During 1911–2011 the main causes of death for men are cancer, infections, and respiratory and cardiovascular disease. With the exception of cancer, there has been a steady fall in all causes of death listed. Respiratory causes peaked in deaths during the 1918 flu epidemic, and then steadily declined; death from infections peaked during both world wars, but generally show a steady decline to a very low rate. Circulatory deaths have shown a steady fall since the 1970s, representing the considerable public health achievement in reducing male smoking. The impact is clearly evident when we consider deaths for men aged 60–4 from heart disease, cancer (predominantly lung cancer), and stroke. There is a considerable decline in male mortality as the cohorts which gave up smoking entered these ages in the 1970s and 1980s. Cancer is interesting as incidence has gone up, probably due to lifestyle, but deaths have gone down, arguably due to modern medicine.

Fleming was transformational in the battle against infections.[18] Vaccination, antimicrobial chemotherapy, and the ability to identify new microbes resulted in a 90 per cent reduction in communicable disease mortality in developed countries.[19] There were significant advances in diagnostic technology, from the discovery of X-rays at the end of nineteenth century through to ECGs and CAT and MRI scans. Geriatric medicine emerged in the mid-twentieth century, with its recognition of the importance of co-morbidities of old age, while the late twentieth century saw the modelling of

DNA (1953) culminating in the human genome project and the science of molecular genetics.[20]

The rise of chronic diseases

As infectious diseases have been reduced, so chronic diseases have increased. This is partly due to lifestyle changes, which may encourage such illnesses as heart disease, diabetes, and some cancers, but also because a higher proportion of the population are now living into older ages where we become more vulnerable to such conditions. Technically, we may describe this process as the *epidemiological transition*,[21] characterized by a reduction in infectious and acute diseases and an increase in chronic and degenerative diseases.

This is seen to comprise four distinct but overlapping stages: an age of pestilence and famine with most people dying before the age of 40; an age of epidemics of infectious diseases with most people surviving to their 50s; an age of chronic disease with life expectancy reaching over 70; and an age of delayed degenerative diseases, with an increase in the age at which individuals succumb to such conditions, a lengthening of the time spent with chronic disease, and a fall in late-life death rates.[22] In advanced economies throughout the twentieth century, there was thus a steady reduction in mortality across the life course resulting in the rectangularization of the life curve, whereby deaths have been consistently pushed further and further back, so that most deaths here now occur after age 80 (Figure 6).

It is now also clear that many of the major health problems associated with this so-called fourth stage are due to personal choice. Individual lifestyle choices are being recognized as modern determinants of morbidity and mortality as individuals increasingly undertake risky behaviour: alcohol, drugs, smoking, unsafe sex, reckless driving, avoiding exercise, and consuming a diet high in

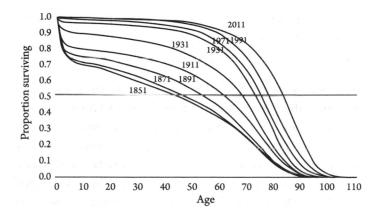

FIG 6 Rectangularization of life curve for England

saturated salt, sugar, and fat. In addition, the increasing prevalence
of neurodegenerative diseases such as Alzheimer's disease and
Parkinson's arise alongside the increase in the numbers of oldest old.

We can also think of this as a process by which death from external causes such as infectious disease, also referred to as exogenous
mortality, is replaced by death from the ageing process, including
most cancers and cardiovascular disease—or endogenous mortality.
This is represented in the so-called rectangularization of the life curve.

Let us consider the past 150 years for England. In 1851, there was
continuous mortality at all ages. Slowly, death was pushed back
later and later, and the line began to form a curve. So much so that
in 1851, less than half the population lived to 45, while currently half
the population can expect to reach their mid 80s.

Mortality in Emerging and Least Developed Economies

As we have seen, in Europe and other advanced economies, the
pace of mortality change was dependent on new ideas and innov-

ations—in sanitation, public health, and nutrition, and then in science, technology, and medicine—to emerge and to diffuse through society. In the emerging economies and least developed economies, these innovations have been transferred from the richer economies and diffused at tremendous speed. Of particular importance have been the widespread vaccination programmes, which by the late twentieth century had spread to the developing countries. In 1970, only 5 per cent of the world's children under five were immunized against measles, tetanus, pertussis ('whooping cough'), diphtheria, and polio; by the 1990s this had increased to around 75 per cent,[23] with the eradication of one of the major child killers—smallpox—by 1979 as one of the great global successes.[24] Developing countries have also benefited from the emergence of well-coordinated international programmes, for example the work of the World Health Organization (WHO), established in 1948, in promoting global vaccination programmes; international famine relief programmes, such as the UN World Food Programme and the Food and Agriculture Organization of the United Nations (FAO); and the emergence of non-governmental organizations working to reduce poverty, famine, and morbidity, for example Water Aid, Oxfam, Save the Children, and UNESCO.

As a result, mortality fell significantly in the latter half of the twentieth century, and life expectancy increased by more than one-third in just 50 years. However, there are still relatively high death rates from infectious diseases, associated with poverty, poor diets, and the limited infrastructure found in least developed economies. Now, alongside these diseases, many such countries are also experiencing a rise in chronic and degenerative diseases.

In summary, we can say that mortality across the life course, arising from exogenous factors such as infectious diseases like malaria and polio, is now coinciding with an increased risk of death from endogenous factors such as cancer which are being exasperated through lifestyle changes, especially unhealthy diet and smoking. Evidence from international epidemiologic research shows that health problems associated with wealthy and aged populations affect a wide and expanding swathe of world population. Over the next 10 to 15 years, people in every world region will suffer more death and disability from non-communicable diseases such as heart disease, cancer, and diabetes than from parasites and infectious diseases.

Yet, despite the considerable increase in chronic disease in middle and low income countries, it is foreseen that there will be a slow convergence in life expectancy. Continued declines in mortality in both the more developed and less developed regions will extend current life expectancy. As Figure 7 reveals, most countries in the less developed world, excluding the least developed countries, now have life expectancies at birth of around 70 years or more. Currently, life expectancy at birth stands at 75 years for males and 81 years for females in the more developed regions, and 67 years for males and 71 years for females in the less developed regions, excluding the least developed countries. These are predicted to reach 81 years (males) and 86 years (females) in the more developed regions, and 76 years (males) and 79.7 years (females) in the less developed regions, excluding the least developed countries by 2050, thereby reducing the gap between these regions (Table 1). However, it is also worth noting that life expectancy in the least developed countries will rise from its current lows of 53 years (males) and 55 years (females) to 71 and 75 years respectively by 2050, a strong closure of the life expectancy gap with the less developed regions as a whole.[25]

The shrinking gap between Latin America and the Caribbean on the one hand, and the Northern American countries on the other

(a) Male

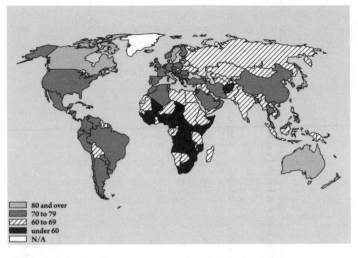

80 and over
70 to 79
60 to 69
under 60
N/A

(b) Female

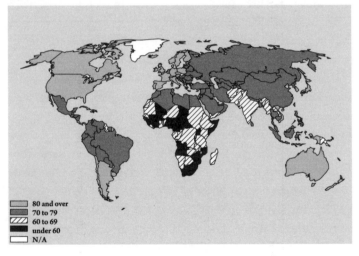

80 and over
70 to 79
60 to 69
under 60
N/A

FIG 7 Life expectancy at birth by country, male and female, 2010–2015

Region	Life expectancy at birth (years)											
	1950–5		2000–5		2030–5		2050–5	
	Male	Female	Male	Female	Male	Female	Male	Female
More developed regions	62.1	67.2	71.9	79.3	78.7	84.1	81.2	86.4
Less developed regions	40.6	42.5	63.7	67.1	71.3	75.3	75.1	78.7
Least developed countries	34.95	37.4	55.1	57.3	66.6	70.1	70.8	74.7
Less developed regions, excluding least developed countries	41.5	43.2	65.5	68.9	72.5	76.5	76.2	79.7

TABLE 1 Life expectancy at birth by region

Country	Life expectancy at birth (years)							
	1950–5		2000–5		2030–5		2050–5	
	Male	Female	Male	Female	Male	Female	Male	Female
UK	66.7	71.8	76.0	80.6	82.3	84.95	85.1	87.3
Italy	64.4	68.1	77.2	83.0	83.7	88.3	86.4	91.0
Mexico	48.9	52.5	72.4	77.4	78.4	82.3	82.8	85.0
Malaysia	53.9	55.8	71.7	76.1	75.5	79.95	79.2	82.6
Niger	35.0	34.9	52.5	52.4	66.6	69.0	70.2	73.3
Somalia	32.5	35.5	49.98	53.1	59.6	63.1	64.5	68.6

TABLE 2 Life expectancy at birth, selected countries

hand, provides a clear example of this convergence. Differences in life expectancy at birth have been reduced considerably for both genders. In the early 1950s, there was a difference of around 17 years for males and 25 years for females. By the beginning of the twenty-first century, these differences had been reduced to just seven years for males and five years for females (Table 2). Much of these improvements are related to a shift from mortality from communicable diseases to mortality from non-communicable diseases.[26]

Childbearing

Jane Austen, the eighteenth-century English novelist, was unmarried and bore no children. However, by the time of her death at 41,[27] probably from either Addison's or Hodgkin's disease,[28] many of her married friends and four of her five sister-in-laws were dead. Childbearing was a perilous activity, with up to ten deaths per 1,000 live births from complications of pregnancy and delivery.[29] In addition, the greater the number of births, the higher the risk of death, with those women giving birth at the time to four or more children facing an up to 50 per cent higher risk of death than women with fewer births.[30] The wife of Jane's brother Edward died two weeks after the birth of her eleventh child, while the wife of her brother Charles went into premature labour and died less than a week after bearing their fourth daughter.[31] At that time, married women bore up to 20 babies, and on average raised seven children. Jane herself was the seventh of eight children and she had 23 surviving nephews and nieces. Jane was briefly engaged to Harris Bigg-Wither before turning him down, and his subsequent wife bore him ten children in the next 18 years.[32] A second failed beau of Jane's, Tom Lefroy, went on to father nine children with his wife. It is not clear that as a married woman Jane Austen would have survived to write *Pride and Prejudice, Mansfield Park, Emma,* or *Persuasion,* or, if she had lived, to have had the intellectual energy to compose such literary works alongside her pregnancy and child rearing.[33]

This was the case for all women. In England and Wales, for example, nearly half of the women who had been born in the early years of the nineteenth century bore six or more live children, around one-quarter between three and five, 13 per cent one or two, and 15 per cent no children. Yet, slowly across the century, fertility rates began to decline. Falling death rates were increasing the number of children who survived and thus had to be supported, and it may be that the decline in infant mortality that was the biggest driver of the reduction of childbearing.[34] In other words, increases in child survival rates reduced the number of births required to achieve the desired number of surviving children.[35] In response, births began to decline, and by the end of the nineteenth century most of Europe's populations were experiencing the beginning of continual fertility decline.[36] Thus, for those women born in the closing decades of the nineteenth century, the proportion of women having six or more children fell to 4 per cent, and those having one or two children rose to 51 per cent.[37]

The decline in European fertility was, however, gradual. In Sweden and England and Wales (countries with good historical statistics), the TFR was between four and five in 1750. It took almost 150 years to drop to three children by 1875, only falling below replacement level in the twentieth century. The fall in childbearing also varied considerably across the continent of Europe, with high levels of fertility being sustained in the east, while in the west of the continent childbearing reached low levels. The story, however, is complex and there is considerable debate over the drivers of child-bearing reduction. In particular, while the desire to reduce disease and death is universal, the wish to reduce childbearing and thus fertility rates is more nuanced. Classical theories, especially from economics, identified economic development, urbanization, and industrialization as the main drivers of mortality and fertility decline. Urban industrial life stripped the family of many of its functions, the growing demand for skilled labour under industrialization, and thus the need for education, increased the costs of children and reduced their potential economic contribution via paid labour, and this resulted in parents lowering fertility to invest more in fewer, healthier children. This therefore explains fertility decline as a response to changing economic systems. However, it is now recognized that economic development is not the only or indeed necessarily the main driver—social factors such as health and education also play a key role.[38] The large European Fertility Project[39] revealed that in some places fertility declined before mortality, while other evidence suggested that it took place along cultural and linguistic, rather than economic, lines.[40]

This may be related in part to the differing ages of first marriage, which were low in Eastern Europe and higher in Northern and Western Europe. France had particularly low levels of childbearing, and fertility fell earlier and faster in rural France than in the economically more developed industrial Britain. Similarly, childbearing rates fell earlier in French-speaking rural Belgium than in Dutch-speaking urban Belgium.[41] Urbanization and industrialization were clearly not the only drivers: cultural, religious, ethnic, and political affiliations were also important factors, as was the use of new birth control methods, which spread out from late eighteenth-century France across the rest of Europe during the following century. While there appears to be little evidence that birth limitation was widespread in pre-industrial England,[42] it appears that from the 1880s an increasing number of women voluntarily limited their fertility, and 'family planning' rapidly became a widely established social norm. Interestingly, however, there is contrasting evidence from both Belgium and France that family planning was occurring some 100 years earlier.[43]

Others argue that fertility decline is driven by social and cultural change, and especially by education.[44] There is a strong association between those countries with a high level of educated women, and those with below replacement fertility levels. Similarly, those countries with low rates of female education have high rates of childbearing. Educating girls in particular encourages later marriage and gives them access to the labour market, which reduces the number of births. Indeed, one of the driving theories behind fertility decline focuses on increased female labour force participation, suggesting that increased female education and autonomy, increased desire for consumption requiring second incomes, and increased female investment in careers have all led to increased female economic activity and subsequent decline in childbearing. Some argue that changes in the 'mindset' of the women and their communities is key, as this enables them to recognize the range of alternative choices they can make, and that transmission of ideas is in fact the biggest factor in declining fertility.[45]

Other cultural theories suggest that fundamental norms and values with regard to the need and desire to have children have changed radically, as societies and their members have become increasingly hedonistic. Thus, self-actualization, freedom of choice, emphasis on quality of life and leisure, and a withdrawal from commitments may all act against the notion of investment in offspring. Recent developments in this area at the micro-level of decision making have drawn on psychological theories to help understand the role of individual psychological traits and how these may determine attitudes to childbearing and family size. It is also clear that the introduction of modern family planning methods has allowed women to choose the number and spacing of births they have.[46] While some contraception has been used in many traditional and historical societies, modern forms of contraception allow more successful family planning.

Declining European fertility…

By the twentieth century, European fertility levels had reached replacement levels, and it was widely thought that they could go no lower. However, apart from a short-lived baby boom in the mid-1960s, fertility moved down from its replacement-level plateau and began a more or less uninterrupted descent to around 1.5 by 2010. By 2015, there was a small spectrum across the region, with the UK and France and the Nordic countries just under replacement, but very low rates of under 1.5 throughout Eastern and Southern Europe.

… goes global

While the European transition was foreseen and monitored, few demographers envisaged that the emerging economies in Asia and Latin America would follow suit, and with such rapidity. In the 1970s to 1990s, the low levels of fertility ranging between 1.3 to 1.8 across Northern and Western Europe and North America were seen as unprecedented and unlikely to continue.[47] In Asia, Latin America, and Africa, TFRs remained high until towards the end of the twentieth century. There was little expectation that fertility would plummet across Asia.[48] While total fertility levels remained low or increased only moderately in Northern and Western Europe and North America, they declined to extremely low levels in

Southern Europe, and—even more unexpectedly—they declined dramatically in Asia, coming down to just above replacement level in the region as a whole, and to very low levels hovering around 1.0 in some countries such as South Korea, Taiwan, Singapore, and the Special Administrative Region of Hong Kong. It should be noted that the speed of fertility transition was much higher in Asia than in Europe. For example, it took Sweden 100 years for the TFR to fall from 4.2 to 3.8 (1800 to 1900), while Bangladesh made the transition from 4.1 to 3.4 in less than 20 years from 1990–5 to 1995–2000.[49]

The promotion of global family planning was given a new thrust in 1969 with the foundation of the United Nations Fund for Population Activities (now the United Nations Population Fund—UNFPA). The number of developing countries with official policies to support family planning rose from just two in 1960 to 115 by 1996. Between 1950 and 2005, fertility in both Asia and Latin America fell from a little under six births per woman to about 2.5 births. The main exceptions are Afghanistan, the Lao People's Democratic Republic, and Pakistan in Asia, and Guatemala, Bolivia, and Paraguay in Latin America. In China, programmes to reduce population growth started in 1972, and in the next seven years fertility fell sharply. In 1979, the one-child policy was enacted and enforced rigorously in urban areas, where fertility fell quickly to one child. China's fertility is currently estimated to be 1.7 births per woman. Childbearing has declined over the past 40 years across the globe from 4.7 in 1970 to 2.5 today (Figure 8). Only in sub-Saharan Africa do TFRs remain high at between four and seven births.[50]

Two-thirds of the world's countries are now at or below replacement level—crudely defined as 2.1 children per woman of childbearing age (Figure 9). These are diverse, including Taiwan, currently the lowest at 1.07 (Hong Kong fell for a while to below

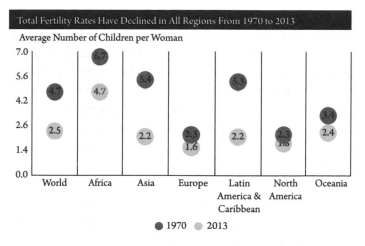

Total Fertility Rates Have Declined in All Regions From 1970 to 2013

Average Number of Children per Woman

| | World | Africa | Asia | Europe | Latin America & Caribbean | North America | Oceania |

● 1970 ● 2013

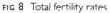

FIG 8 Total fertility rates

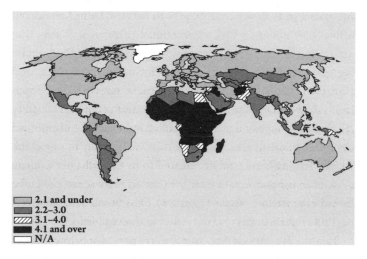

2.1 and under
2.2–3.0
3.1–4.0
4.1 and over
N/A

FIG 9 Total fertility, 2005–10 (children per woman)

1 at 0.99 in 2012 and now stands at 1.2, while Macao is 1.19), Thailand, Vietnam, Mauritius, Iran, Chile, Poland, Barbados, Germany, and the US. A further 50 are low-medium, with a TFR of 2.1 to 3 children. These include India, Botswana, Bangladesh, Indonesia, Argentina, Mexico, Venezuela, and South Africa. Twenty-seven are at high-medium levels of 3 to 4.1—including Zimbabwe, Egypt, and Pakistan. However, 43 still have high levels of 4.1 and above— most but not all are in sub-Saharan Africa, and most are classified by the UN as least developed economies. Here, women are on average still bearing 5.2 children, with Niger having the highest TFR at 7.6.

Future Challenges

As we discussed in Chapter 1, the major challenges which arise in all regions from these demographic shifts are how to sustain and enhance well-being across an individual's life, while at the same time reducing the inequalities within each generation and ensuring an equitable reallocation of resources between the generations. The different drivers of mortality and fertility change are causing an age-structural change across the globe. But there are also specific challenges which arise from extreme population change. In particular, we may identify four main challenges which are affecting different parts of the world: very low fertility in many parts of Europe and increasingly in some Asian countries; continued high fertility, especially in sub-Saharan Africa; continued high rates of morbidity and mortality in the least developed economies; and the implications of ever-increasing longevity and the growth of the oldest old population, currently in advanced economies, but set to spread to the emerging economies during this century.

Very low fertility

In 1950, Europe's TFR was 2.5 children per reproductive woman. This had fallen to 1.5 by 2010. Future fertility is difficult to predict: projected TFRs are between 1.34 and 2.34 children per woman by 2045.[51] Alongside the well-recognized low fertility of Eastern Europe and the southern Mediterranean countries standing below 1.5, we see a similar pattern emerging in Asia. Singapore, Hong Kong, and South Korea have now fallen to below 1.25, while Taiwan has the lowest TFR in the world. Some demographers have expressed concern that due to *demographic inertia*, a very low fertility rate could become irreversible.[52]

Some demographers now argue that low-fertility countries are in the midst of a *second demographic transition* which is keeping fertility well below replacement. This may be due to technological advances and changes in the labour market, which have altered the costs and rewards of marriage and child rearing.[53] Others suggest it may be ideational changes which have accompanied our increased affluence, leading to a focus on individual autonomy and self-realisation.[54] In particular, the evolutionary link between the sex drive and procreation has clearly been broken through the introduction of modern contraception, and reproduction is now merely a function of individual preferences and culturally determined norms.[55]

Indeed, some Asian and European countries may well be in a so-called *low fertility trap*[56] which arises both through demographic factors (the fact that fewer potential mothers in the future will result in fewer births) and sociological ones (ideal family size for the younger generations is declining as a consequence of the lower childbearing they see in previous generations). Here it is argued that countries with very low childbearing rates of below 1.5 for more than one generation become adapted to childless or one-child families, and it is then very difficult to raise fertility again.[57] Employment patterns change, childcare and schools are reduced, and there is a shift from a family/child orientated society to an individualistic society, with children part of individual fulfilment and well-being. There is a typical sequence of events leading to below replacement fertility: a move from marriage to cohabitation, with the nuclear family being replaced by a complex array of family structures; and an emphasis on children as enhancing parental well-being, with childlessness also viewed as a positive means of adult personal fulfilment. Contraception comes to be viewed not just as a means to reduce family size and thus enhance family well-being, but also to enhance personal well-being. This leads to societies of individually orientated people striving for the successful combination of family life, lifestyle consumption, and employment which now defines adulthood. Childlessness or one-child families become the norm, and the rationale for fertility control moves from the well-being of the family unit to the self-fulfilment of the individual. Germany provides a good case example here (Figure 10 and Table 3).

Low fertility in former West Germany is largely attributable to high childlessness, especially among tertiary educated women.[58] This also appears to be the case in China. Here, the one-child policy, which was initiated in 1980, has been in place for over 30 years, and there is now a large number of one-child children who are of childbearing age. Despite the fact that they are allowed two children, survey evidence suggests that many are choosing to have just one child themselves. Is this because it is their own experience growing up in a society of one-child families. A 2012 study in Shanghai, for example, reported that fewer than 10 per cent of those now eligible to have more than one child had actually done so,[59] as exemplified by the following case study.

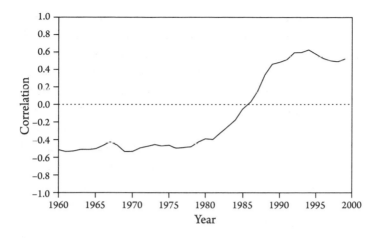

FIG 10 Correlation between fertility (TFR) and rate of female labour force participation in OECD countries

Yin San, a 36-year-old mother working for an international company, is an example of a modern Chinese mother able to have a second child but hesitant to do so. She would like to ensure that her 3-year-old daughter, YiYi, is given every advantage, and this is expensive. YiYi has attended extra classes since she was eight months old. Yin has enrolled YiYi in a bilingual kindergarten, and in addition pays for her to have private swimming lessons, with drawing, music, and ballet lessons planned for the future. Yin feels that such a broad education is essential to succeed in modern-day China.[60]

This position is backed up by studies of voluntarily stated fertility preferences which have found a growing desire among parents in both rural and urban areas of China to have just one child.[61] The greater challenge going forward, however, may be with regard to how low fertility rates will fall. We shall return to the implications of this in Chapter 3.

Period	1970–5	1975–80	1980–5	1985–90	1990–5	1995–2000	2000–5	2005–10
Total fertility	1.71	1.51	1.46	1.43	1.3	1.35	1.35	1.36

TABLE 3 TFR, Germany

United Nations (2015) *World Population Prospects: The 2015 Revision*. Population Division of the Department of Economic and Social Affairs of the United Nations Secretariat, New York. Accessed 17 November 2015. With permission.

Continued high fertility

While fertility is falling in both advanced and emerging economies, it still remains high in the least developed economies, most of which are found in sub-Saharan Africa. With the UN 2012 population revision predicting a further billion people on the planet, leading to a population of 11 billion by the end of this century, attention has again turned to the plight of Africa, where the majority of the extra billion are predicted to be born over the coming decades.

Drawing on experience from other developing countries, it was expected that the decline in infant and child mortality in sub-Saharan Africa would be followed by a decline in fertility to around replacement level. However, the pace of fertility decline in sub-Saharan Africa is weak compared to other regions,[62] and there is some evidence of stalling in the rate of decline in childbearing.[63] Recent surveys of these stalling fertility declines have identified that the region of sub-Saharan Africa that lies north of Botswana and Namibia stands out from the rest of the developing world,[64] and almost two-thirds of the countries in the region experienced no significant fertility decline in the first decade of the twenty-first century. The position of Kenya illustrates this.[65] The number of children per woman of childbearing age dropped dramatically in the last three decades of the twentieth century, falling from over eight in 1970 to five by 2000. However, since then TFR has remained at just below five. Similarly, Benin, Rwanda, and Zambia have declined little in recent years.[66] In the southern African countries,[67] on the other hand, fertility has fallen below four children per woman.

There is currently a debate as to whether these stalls in Africa are but a minor pause in the course of the fertility decline, or whether this is an indication of deeper processes.[68] In particular, it may be that a fertility rate above replacement is embedded in the culture of sub-Saharan society, and that desired family size is higher than the two-child norm found in most other parts of the world.[69] Even if childbearing does begin to decline again in these countries, given the large young populations living there, if the stalls last for several years or even decades they could have serious consequences for long-term population growth, especially as they are occurring at such relatively high levels of childbearing. The near 10 per cent projected increase in maximum global population this century largely arises from the fact that the fertility rate in Africa has declined more slowly than expected, and appears to be stalling in several countries. The UN medium population growth scenario is that TFR in sub-Saharan Africa will fall to three children per woman by 2050. If this occurs, then the African population will increase from almost 1 billion to 2.5 billion by 2050 and 4.4 billion by 2100. However, if the regional reduction in childbearing stalls and remains at its current level of 5.5, then sub-Saharan Africa's population will be approaching 2 billion by 2050 and some 4 billion by the end of the century.

The challenge here is clear: when high fertility is combined with relatively low mortality, it leads to rapid population growth and high rates of child dependency.[70] Furthermore, continuing high fertility delays the prospect of a demographic dividend arising from declining dependency rates,[71] undermines the prospects for economic and social development, and makes it more difficult for households to escape from poverty. We shall consider this further in Chapter 5.

High morbidity and mortality

While there have been significant advances in reducing mortality in middle and low income countries, many of these still lag behind the progress seen in advanced economies.[72] Of particular concern is infant mortality. On average for OECD countries, this has fallen to eight per 1,000, but it is still some 100 per 1,000 in many of the least developed economies. While vaccination programmes have made huge inroads into reducing death from infectious diseases,[73] 2.4 per cent of children in Asia and 22.5 per cent[74] in Africa still die from malaria. Diarrhoeal diseases account for 14.6 per cent of deaths among children under five in Africa and 20.6 per cent in South East Asia. Similarly, contaminated water and poor sanitation still account for high mortality rates especially among the under fives. It is estimated that this leads to some 1.7 million deaths a year globally, mainly through infectious diarrhoea, 90 per cent of these being deaths of children.[75]

A similar picture emerges from poor nutrition. Half of childhood deaths in developing countries arise from under nutrition. Underweight children are at increased risk of mortality from infectious illnesses such as diarrhoea and pneumonia. Globally, some 100 million children under five, around 16 per cent, are underweight; one-third of the under fives in South Asia, some 60 million; and one-fifth in sub-Saharan Africa, reaching 30 million.[76] Over one-quarter of African children are 'stunted'. In other words, due to extreme malnourishment their bodies and brains fail to develop properly—this is an irreversible condition affecting them for life. According to Harper et al., 'Chronic poverty has serious consequences for children, not least the strong likelihood of suffering a premature death from easily preventable health problems, or lifelong ill health due to deprivations.'[77] In addition, these economies still experience high levels of infant and maternal mortality.

Furthermore, many of these economies are also experiencing a rise in chronic and degenerative diseases. The burden of chronic

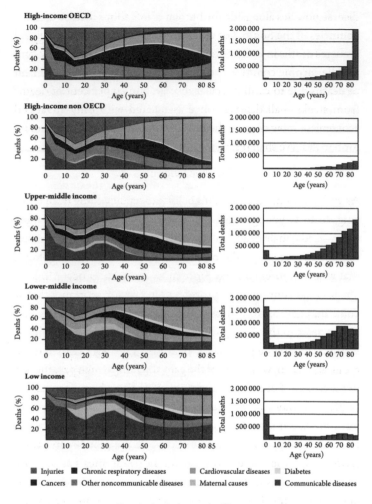

FIG 11 Female deaths across the life course, 2012

disease now lies alongside the burden of infectious disease in many countries of the South. For example, of the some 1.5 million global diabetes deaths in 2012, more than 80 per cent occurred in low- and middle-income countries; 70 per cent of cancer deaths, 82 per cent of deaths due to cardiovascular disease, and 89 per cent of deaths from stroke—all diseases once associated with only advanced economies—now occur in these less developed economies (Figure 11) for females. We shall return to this in Chapter 5.

Extreme longevity

As we have seen, the early gains in life expectancy came from reducing death at younger ages—in particular infant and child mortality—and female deaths in childbirth. With every year that passes, there is an increase in the proportion of successive birth cohorts that reaches retirement age. Since most deaths now occur in later life, it is the continuing improvement in late-life mortality that is contributing most to increasing life expectancy at birth. Over the last 20 years in the United Kingdom, male life expectancy at birth has increased by 5.6 years, i.e. at an average rate of more than three months per year, with most of the gain accruing to men past the age of retirement. Four of those additional life years have been added to life expectancy at the age of 65. Death rates in older men have not only fallen sharply in this time—by almost one-half in the 60–9 age group and one-third in the 70–9 age group—and from relatively high levels, but the decline in death rates has actually been *accelerating*, which accounts for the more or less linear increase in life expectancy. The average annual rate of improvement between 2000 and 2005 was twice as high as it was in the late 1980s. Death rates among older women have followed a similar trend, though the gains have been not quite so large.

In the United States, the gains in life expectancy over the past few decades have been more modest than in most other OECD countries.[78] Over the last 20 years, US male life expectancy at birth has increased by 4.6 years, with 2.6 of those additional life years being added to life expectancy at the age 65.[79]

Death rates in older men have fallen by almost 40 per cent in the 65–74 age group and 30 per cent in the 75–84 age group. Gains have not been quite as large among older women—around one-quarter in the 65–74 age group and almost one-fifth in 75–84 age group. Between 2003 and 2013, the US population aged 55–64 grew from 28 to 39 million. In 2003, the 55–64 age group accounted for 9.7 per cent of the population; by 2013, this share had increased to 12.4 per cent. By 2030, the 55–64 age group will likely decrease to 10.8 per cent as the baby boomers pass through this age group and swell the ranks of the 65–74 and 75–84 age groups.[80]

A key set of questions thus revolve around whether increases in both life expectancy and in life extension or longevity will continue. In other words, will there be an increase in average years lived by humans and also maximum years attained by human beings? And will life expectancy increase in line with life extension? In other words, will we all enjoy the benefits of longevity or will it only be for a few?

Life expectancy and life extension are often confused but are two distinct concepts. In general terms, *life expectancy* refers to the average number of years individuals within a population can expect to live. In technical terms, life expectancy is the average number of additional years a person would live *if current mortality conditions applied*. This caveat is important and explains why current life expectancy for women in the UK is 82, and yet the Office of National Statistics announced in 2014 that the first UK cohort[81] of baby girls had been born with a life expectancy of 100. Indeed, the life expectancy of babies born in many advanced economies in the early twenty-first century is probably around 103. This is because across the lifetime of these baby girls the current death rates will change considerably, and they will benefit from this. Most of their lives, therefore, they will not be living under the current mortality conditions. Increases in life expectancy are driven to a large extent by falls in mortality at younger ages, as more infants, children, and young people survive so the average life expectancy of the population is increased. In advanced economies, life expectancy has been increasing by two and a half years per decade for the past 150 years, or six hours per day.

Life extension is the pushing back of the maximum number of years a human population can reach. Humans have evolved to live long enough to reproduce and ensure the survival of their offspring. This is the *essential life span*. But in most countries of the world, most of us live well beyond this essential life span. In advanced economies, the greatest falls in mortality are now being experienced in later life, among the oldest old. The drivers of life extension appear to be fourfold: healthy living, disease prevention and cure, age retardation or senescence prevention, and regenerative medicine. It has been argued that healthy living and disease prevention and cure can push the length of most lives in advanced economies to 100 years. Indeed, centenarians in the UK are likely to increase from around 12,000 currently to around half a million by the middle of the century and 1 million by the end.[82] Eight million people currently alive in the UK are likely to reach a century, 50 million in Europe. The life expectancy of babies born today is predicted to be around 103 in the UK, 104 in the US, and 107 in Japan (see Table 4).[83] However, we shall probably

	2000	2001	2002	2003	2004	2005	2006	2007
Canada	102	102	103	103	103	104	104	104
Denmark	99	99	100	100	101	101	101	101
France	102	102	103	103	103	104	104	104
Germany	99	100	100	100	101	101	101	102
Italy	102	102	102	103	103	103	104	104
Japan	104	105	105	105	106	106	106	107
UK	100	101	101	101	102	102	103	103
US	101	102	102	103	103	103	104	104

TABLE 4 Oldest age at which at least 50 per cent of a birth cohort is still alive in eight countries

Reprinted from The Lancet, Vol. 374, Christensen, K., Doblhammer, G., Rau, R., and Vaupel, J. W, 'Ageing Populations: The Challenges Ahead', 1196–202, Copyright 2009, with permission from Elsevier.

need age retardation and regenerative medicine to achieve real life extension.

Will increases in life expectancy be accompanied by increases in life extension or are we seeing a compression of longevity after 100? In other words, will the predicted increases in centenarians over the coming century be accompanied by increases in super-centenarians, those aged over 110? The relevant evidence here can be drawn from deaths among the oldest old—those over 80. Late-life mortality rates in many developed countries are declining and currently show no signs of slowing. If we take not life expectancy but 'modal age at death'—in other words, the age each year at which most people in the population die—in countries such as Japan (where we have sufficient numbers of old people to study this), we find that the mode is some six years older than the average; and importantly, as the mode increases so the tail—or the distribution of deaths above this mode—is also sliding to higher ages. We call this a 'shifting mortality scenario' and this provides evidence—at least for Japan—that as we see an increase in centenarians so we should expect to see an increase in super-centenarians.

However, in order to continue these extreme longevity increases, we may have to address senescence—or ageing—itself. For while some argue that increases in life extension will continue,[84] others such as bio-demographers Jay Olshansky and Bruce Carnes, maintain that we need biological intervention to continue the trends.[85] Discussion of the implications of this is continued in Chapter 3.

Age-structural challenges

These then are the challenges arising from the specific demographic drivers we are experiencing in the twenty-first century. All will lead to a shift in the age structure, but this will be played out differently in different regions. Advanced economies thus face the general ageing of their populations due to very low fertility and continued falling mortality rates among those in later life, and especially the oldest old. However, these economies have had time to plan for this age-structural shift, which has moved slowly over the past two centuries. This is unlike the challenge facing emerging economies, which are undergoing a rapid change in the age structure of their populations. Dramatically falling fertility rates and steadily falling mortality rates are changing their population structures in a matter of decades, requiring a rapid response to the different needs and demands of the expanding and contracting age groups. In contrast, many economies in sub-Saharan Africa appear still to be sitting on the cusp of the fertility transition, with possibly stalling fertility fall, and the cultural acceptance of relatively high childbearing in relation to the rest of the world. Alongside a variety of development concerns, these economies also face the challenges that large proportions of dependent infants and children may ultimately bring to modernizing economies and societies. It is to these specific population challenges we shall now turn.

CHAPTER THREE

The Grey Burden

Growing national debt since 2008 has focused government attention on two apparently conflicting priorities: the need to sustain
public spending on pensions and health care versus the need to
reduce budget deficits. This shift from predominantly young to
predominantly older populations has both broad macro-economic
implications as well as important financial consequences for both
the public and private sector. Put this together with the global financial crisis and you have the perfect storm of disruption to national
economies.[1]

As we saw in Chapter 2, different regions of the world are experiencing the age shift in different ways and magnitudes. In addition,
each is also currently challenged by a particular set of demographic
dynamics which are controlling the pace and form of the change.
Advanced economies are well along the way of the age-structural
shift, which has been in progress for a couple of hundred years
since the start of the demographic transition in Europe in the mid-
eighteenth century. Alongside the general mass ageing of their
populations, with a steady increase in both the mean and median
ages and in average life expectancy, they are also facing the challenge of extreme low fertility, and low mortality rates among the
oldest old. While the first is changing their worker to dependent

ratio, the second is challenging the ability to care for the large numbers in and approaching extreme frailty.

The rhetoric and reality of the age-structural change facing advanced economies are often confused:

- 'Ageing: Europe's growing problem.' BBC Business News, September 2002.
- 'Ageing in Europe...has been one of the most remarkable success stories of our time.' United Nations Economic Commission for Europe, April 2002.
- Global ageing is a 'threat more grave and certain than those posed by chemical weapons, nuclear proliferation, or ethnic strife'. US Secretary of Commerce, Peterson, 1999.
- 'People should be paid to have more children.' Edmund Stoiber, German Christian Social Union leader, January 2001.
- 'Too many people: Europe's population problem' Optimum Population Trust, 2005.

Most advanced economies have aged continuously over the past century. By 2030, nearly half the population of Western Europe (44.7 per cent) will be over 50, one-quarter over 65, and 12.7 per cent over 75. As discussed in Chapter 2, longevity has increased, and it is now forecast that the real life expectancy of today's European babies will be well over 100 years, with over 5 million centenarians alive in Europe by the end of the twenty-first century. This will clearly have significant implications for labour supply, family and household structure, health and welfare service demand, patterns of saving and consumption, provision of housing and transport, leisure and community behaviour, and networks and social interaction. As governments and policymakers have awakened to the implications of population ageing, so the demographic burden hypothesis has spread. National health services, and even economies, are predicted to collapse under the strain of health and pension demand, and families will no longer be there to compensate for failing public provision.

Japan is often seen as the classic ageing society. Japan's rapid fertility decline in the post-Second World War period brought its childbearing levels to the lowest in the world—reaching replacement in the late 1950s, it fell to 1.5 in the 1990s and further to 1.30 in 2005, recovering slightly to its current TFR of 1.40. Japan also led the world in its mortality decline, with male life expectancy rising from around 50 in the immediate post-war years to 69 by the mid-1960s, and female life expectancy rising from 54 to 74. Life expectancies in Japan are now some of the highest in the world at 80 for men and 86 for women. Late-life life expectancy is even higher, with male life expectancy at 60 now 23, and for women 28. Building on the rapid post-Second World War recovery, Japan established universal pension and health care systems. Initially based on a large accumulated reserve fund, Japan had to shift to a pay-as-you-go system in 1985.[2] More recently in 2004, the government introduced a system of fixed contributions and reduced benefits to secure the future stability of the scheme in the light of extreme ageing. Even so, the social security system now faces serious financing problems, as the number of beneficiaries is increasing at a time when the working population is declining—a simultaneous increase in payments and decrease in revenues. In a similar move, the government has also now introduced a system of long-term care insurance in an attempt to curb the upward spiralling of medical care costs.

The US is also facing considerable budget deficits, in part due to its public social security and health programmes. Future scenarios predict that the deficit will range from between 8 per cent and 20 per cent of GDP by 2050. The UK is in a different situation as there has been a continuous shift towards the older individual bearing the financial responsibility of health and pension costs, but even here the government has raised the state pension age to 66 from 2016 in a direct move to cut the UK budget deficit by some £13 billion a year. And Australia—currently experiencing annual surpluses—faces a budget deficit of $100 billion Australian dollars in ten years' time, around 4 per cent of GDP, of which $30 billion dollars will arise from increased health care spending. The current Liberal government wishes to increase the state pension age (Age Pension age) from 2017 until it reaches the age of 70 years in 2035, affecting the 1966 birth cohort onwards.

The International Monetary Fund in particular highlighted the costs associated with future population ageing and the movement of Europe's post-war bulge through the population structure, suggesting for example that former Eastern European economies would acquire an accumulated deficit of well over 50 per cent of GDP over the next 50 years, raising the spectre of a 'meltdown of pension systems'.[3] For further robust data on pensions and economic costs of ageing populations in these regions, there are several good websites which are kept up to date by organizations such as the World Bank[4] and *The Economist*.[5]

Yet the major concerns—public spending on pensions, high dependency ratios between workers and non-workers, increases in health care costs, declining availability of family based care, and a slowdown in consumption due to an increase in older people and a decrease in younger people—are based on assumptions developed from the characteristics and behaviours of current older populations. Some of these fears are supported by evidence, but many are speculative myths, widespread in public debate but lacking a robust evidential base. Behind the rhetoric defining dependency and productivity lies the complexity of social and economic behaviour and the ability of societies and individuals to adapt to changing circumstances. It is highly likely that future generations of older adults will have higher levels of human capital—in terms of education, skills, and abilities—and that old age, as defined by retirement and dependency, will occur at far older ages than currently. In addition, these are all issues which can be addressed by policy, given the political and economic will.

The challenge for advanced economies is that not only are individuals living longer, they are doing so within a population which is itself growing older. As we discussed in Chapter 1, to grow old in a society where most people are young is fundamentally different from doing so in a society where most people are old. Young nations have high proportions of economically active individuals with the potential to produce the wealth needed to support dependents, both old and young. However, old populations have a lower proportion of workers, and thus the responsibility of providing for old age dependency may increasingly fall to the older people themselves. In addition, societies with a large proportion of their populations in old age have to consider how to redistribute resources away from a focus on younger people towards older people in an equitable manner, both intergenerationally (between the generations) and intragenerationally (within each generation). The major challenges for advanced economies are framed by increasing decline and dependency within the population, inequalities, and equitable redistribution of resources.

Production into consumption

As we discussed in Chapter 1, with the percentage of individuals within each age group shifting as we move through the twenty and twenty-first centuries, so a wave-like bulge forms across the population structure, flowing over time from a large percentage of young dependents or children, through a large percentage of workers, to a large percentage of older dependents. The redistribution of resources through the generations is linked to the economic life-cycle and may be described as the *generational economy*.[6] This comprises the intergenerational distribution of income or consumption which results from the institutions and mechanisms used by each generation to produce, consume, share, and save resources; the economic flow between different generations; and the contract which governs this.

Across our lives, an individual typically undertakes four different sets of economic activities: producing, consuming, saving, and sharing. As we saw in Chapter 1, during an individual's prime working years, he or she will typically produce more than they consume. Consumption takes place across the life cycle, and can be consumption of goods or services. Sharing may be publicly via taxation, which funds education, health care, and pensions for example, or privately within families and households. Saving allows assets accumulated at one stage of the life cycle to be used at a later stage, as in paying off a housing loan or creating a retirement pension.

In order for standards of living to be sustained, those who are working must generate sufficient resources to fund their own material needs; to transfer resources to both young and old dependents; and to provide for their own future dependency in old age. This is where the changing support ratios of aging populations become important, because the proportion of producers to dependents declines as a society reaches the late stage of the demographic transition. One of the key issues in advanced economies is that while in traditional societies older people continued to produce well into old age, in modern societies people after retirement consume more than they produce. This consumption takes the form of pensions, health and long-term care, and the drawdown of assets.

That is not to say that older people have not 'earned' this drawdown through earlier taxation, pension contributions, and the careful housekeeping of their assets, nor to ignore their contribution through unpaid and often unrecorded care, but to note that in a population with a large proportion of retired adults, this will have an economic impact.

It is argued that the economic boom experienced by Japan in the 1960s was related to its demographic dividend. Economic calculations[7] suggest that Japan's proportion of producers grew consistently from the end of the Second World War until the 1980s, mirroring the rise of the demographic dividend, and outstripping the proportion of consumers in the population. However, from the 1990s onwards Japan's ageing population took centre stage; having experienced a fourfold increase in the percentage of the population aged over 65 in 55 years (5 per cent in 1950 to 20 per cent by 2005) and with limited immigration, its population also started to decline in size. As is clear from Japan, the context to the economic challenge is the age-structural change in the population, or the changing composition of ages within a population.

Elderly dependency

In Chapter 1, the concept of the *support ratio*—the ratio of workers to consumers—was introduced. Another way of formulating this is the relationship of dependents, young and old, to workers—the *dependency ratio*.[8] These comprise *elderly dependency ratios* (EDRs), the number of persons of working age (aged 15 to 64) per person aged 65 or over; *youth dependency ratios* (YDRs), the number of persons of working age (aged 15 to 64) per person aged 15 or under; and *total dependency ratios* (TDRs), the number of those aged 15 to 64 compared with those outside this age range. The shift in TDR from youth dependency to elderly dependency may be a useful measure in determining when a population reaches demographic maturity.

If we consider these different dependency ratios, the next decades will see a rapid shift towards increased EDR in most industrialized countries. Europe as a region will be most affected: the average EDR for the 25 members of the European Union (EU25) as a whole is expected to double as the working-age population (15 to 64 years) decreases by 48 million between now and 2050.[9] The EU25 will thus change from having four to only two persons of working age for each citizen aged 65 and above, or an EDR of 50;100. However, there will be considerable variations even here. Several European countries have already gone through significant population ageing, and those countries which are already demographically old—Belgium, France, the Netherlands, Norway, Denmark, Sweden, and the United Kingdom—are projected to see relatively small increases in dependency ratios over the next 40 years. European EDRs will be highest in Italy, Spain, Greece, and Germany[10] where childbearing rates are very low.

Germany provides another example of an extreme aged society. Though one nation now, its demographic history cannot be disconnected from its political past. Thus, the eastern and western parts of the country experienced different fertility and mortality rates, and this is still reflected today. Following unification, the TFR of former East Germany reached 0.77, and has only recently increased to its current level of 1.46, with former West Germany at 1.38. As a consequence, population ageing has progressed faster in the east of the country, encouraged further by strong flows of young outmigration to the west. There is expected to be a fall in the national population level over the coming decades as well as a shrinkage of the labour force from its current 55 million to under 40 million by the middle of the century. Despite unification, the institutions of the past still influence the position of the population today. For example, in the east 100 per cent of pensioners' income comes from the public purse, as opposed to only 80 per cent in the west; similarly in the east of the country, there is still a strong tradition of unemployment benefits for those older workers out of employment prior to retirement, with around one-fifth taking them in the east, and only 8 per cent in the west.

Let's question the assumptions

Clearly these concerns are based on a series of assumptions, and it is worth considering them more closely. The assumptions may be positioned within two broad debates. First, the population context of the current demographic drivers is affected by policies and institutions—and it is these and not the demographics themselves which frame the outcomes. We need to recognize the impact of current institutions—and in particular to recognize that twenty-first-century living is structured by twentieth-century institutions which may not be effective for twenty-first-century dynamics. Second, there are preconceptions around the economic contribution of older adults and their productivity which are not supported by robust evidence, and these need to be revisited. It is these institutions and public perceptions which influence the behaviour of individuals in these societies.[11]

Institutional frameworks

As the ageing of the population in advanced economies became apparent, so these economies moved to establish institutions to address the future challenges. Pension systems and long-term care systems now exist across the developed world. However, these institutions may facilitate higher dependency ratios or larger transfers across the generations. Generous public pension systems allow healthy, active, and potentially productive individuals to retire, and then expect to be supported in this retirement for up to 40 years. Or societies which discriminate on stereotypical grounds against older workers, increasingly defined as over 50, and encourage them to withdraw from economic activity up to 40 years before the expected end of their lives.

Figure 12 illustrates the average years men lived after retirement in 1970 and in 2004, for selected economies. The most extreme case is France, where life expectancy on retirement doubled from 11 to 22 years over the three decades, not due to increases in life expectancy alone, but a combination of increasingly early retirement as life expectancy increased.

It has also been suggested, for example, that pension incentives are an important influence on early withdrawal from economic activity, and may explain differences in continued employment across economies on the basis of state pension incentives.[12] Studies

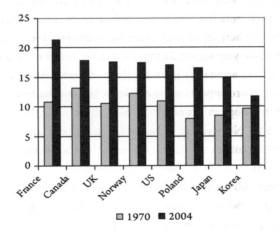

FIG 12 Life expectancy at actual age of retirement in 1970 and 2004

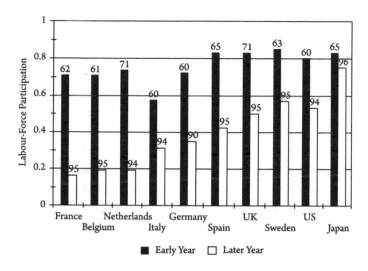

FIG 13 Decline in labour force participation, age 60–4

by the US economists, Gruber and Wise, find that exits from employment were lower in the US than in Germany and France, where there was less financial incentive to continue (Figure 13). However, others argue that individuals are not able to calculate their year-by-year accumulation of social security wealth, and even less likely to accurately estimate their life expectancies. Clearly, however, there appears to be a pattern between early retirement in those European economies with built-in incentives to retire (France, the Netherlands, Italy, and Germany) and later retirement in those countries where the incentive is less (Sweden, the US, and Japan).

In particular, the institutional framework facilitates the relationship between production and consumption in a country. A comparison between Germany and the US provides a good example here. Germany is considered to be the oldest welfare state in the world, with social insurance from the 1890s. The needs of the dependent age groups are publically funded, with a large proportion of the nation's GDP spent on providing health, education, and pensions. Currently, schools are publically financed and free for all students, with around 98 per cent of young people attending free state schools.[13] At the other end of the life cycle, the German pension system commenced in 1889 with a retirement age of 70, based on a capital-funded system. After the economic devastation of the Depression and two world wars, it was reorganized as a pay-as-you-go system in 1957, with a high wages-to-pension replacement level, and the allowance of early retirement from the 1970s.[14] While this has recently been tightened up, pensions still account for over 10 per cent of German GDP:[15] 85 per cent of the workforce is covered by the public sector pension scheme, and 80 per cent of pensioner income comes from the public pension. The average age of retirement is 61, but there is high unemployment among those over age 50. In addition, Germany has a publically financed healthcare system, covering nearly 90 per cent of the population. Under the German system, young people spend a long period of time in the free education system at one end of the life cycle, while early retirement schemes, sound pension provision, plus good unemployment benefits for older workers encourage early exit from the labour market at the other end of the life cycle.[16]

Consumption of publically funded goods is thus high among the dependent young and old, while the time spent in production via the economic labour market is relatively low (Figure 14). Our understanding of this has been significantly increased through the recent work on National Transfer Accounts.[17] As an average, Germans are economically productive between 27 and 57, for 30 years within an ever-lengthening life. It is now recognized that the sustainability of the system is under threat, and the German

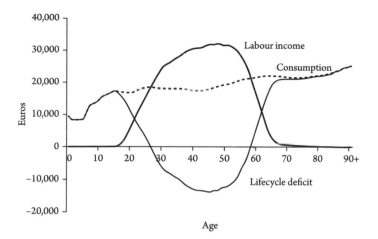

FIG 14 Per capita labour income, consumption, and the lifecycle deficit: Germany, 2003

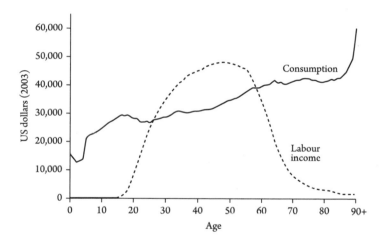

FIG 15 Total consumption (private plus public) and labour income: United States, 2003

government is looking for solutions, including the lengthening of the working life.

Compare this with the situation of the US (Figure 15). Here we see that while old-age consumption is high, so is old-age productivity. The US pension system—Social Security[18]—was introduced in 1935. It has more than 90 per cent coverage, with an average replacement rate of 40 per cent, low by European standards. The US has no universal public health care system. However, those over 65 are covered by the publically funded Medicare system, while poor older people qualify under the Medicaid system for nursing home care. The US runs a mixed public/private education system at all levels, with just over 10 per cent of school age students and over 20 per cent of tertiary age students attending private institutions. At the other end of the life cycle, while the twentieth century saw a decline in older workers, with the median age at male retirement falling from over 80 at the turn of the century to 63 at the end, this was still high in relation to other advanced economies, and during the early years of the twenty-first century it has risen again to 65. There are various explanations for this high retention of older workers. However, the growing educational ability of successive cohorts entering later working ages has been important in maintaining their employability. In addition, the US was one of the first countries to introduce age discrimination legislation for those aged between 40 and 65 in 1967; for those up to age 70 in 1978; and without an upper age limit in 1986.[19]

What is clear from Figure 16 is the growing levels of consumption across the life course, with a dramatic increase in old age. By age 80, consumption is 50 per cent higher than at 20, and by age 90 it is more than double that at 25. As Figure 16 reveals, it is the massive cost of late-life health care, and in particular long-term care, which has been responsible for this dramatic increase in late-life

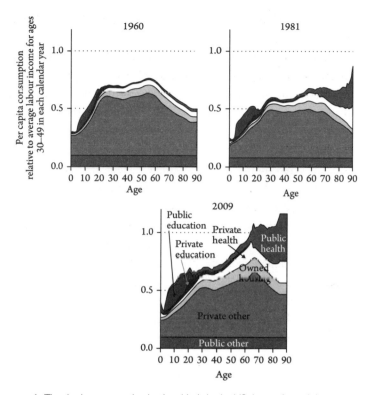

FIG 16 The rise in consumption by the elderly in the US since 1960, and the growing role of public transfers to the elderly

consumption in recent years, with both public and private spending significantly growing in these areas. In 1960, consumption declined after age 60, and public and private spending on both education and health were quite limited. During the 1960s, new public programmes were introduced to pay for health care,[20] and by the 1970s public pension benefits had become more generous. The impact of both of these can be seen in the 1981 graph, with the increased spending on health care and an increase in private consumption at older ages as the increased pension benefits enter the system. By 2007, the age profile of consumption rose very sharply, beginning with education and continuing towards the 1990s when spending on long-term care increased considerably.

However, of equal significance is the long time spent in economic employment in the US. Unlike the German case, economically productive life in the US runs for many from their late teens to their 70s.

Producing, consuming, and paying taxes

Much of the concern around the economic challenge arises from the presumption that future older labour forces will be less productive and less innovative, and that an older population will consume less—both with negative consequences for economies. However, in the advanced economies at least, new cohorts of highly educated, skilled, and increasingly healthy populations are approaching traditional retirement ages and are increasingly remaining in economic activity—producing, consuming, and paying taxes. Furthermore, longer lives allow a great accumulation of assets which, when invested, can enhance productivity, generate asset income, and raise living standards. Similarly, while population ageing may affect the aggregate savings rate by raising the fraction of the population in age groups traditionally associated with drawdown, it may also affect an economy's average level of savings per capita, as individuals approaching and shortly after retirement tend to have higher levels of savings than those at the start of their working career. It has been estimated, for example, that the US will see a 25 per cent increase in national net worth per person of working age by the middle of the century due to population ageing alone. Similarly, it has been argued that increased life expectancies can be expected to induce increased savings over the working life in order to finance a continued high standard of living in retirement.[21] These two factors—the need to save more for a longer retirement and the changes in the age distribution of a population—have the potential to raise the asset income of a nation.

The second demographic dividend

Interest in the advanced economies is thus now turning to the possibility of a second demographic dividend. As we discussed in Chapter 2, as societies transition from largely rural agrarian economies with high fertility and mortality rates to urban industrial ones, mortality and then fertility rates fall. The low proportion of young child dependents and still low proportion of older dependents ensures a high percentage of those of working age who, given the right circumstances, are able to invest their productivity in economic growth. This is the first demographic dividend and will be discussed in more detail in Chapter 4. After a few decades, low fertility rates ensure that the number of young workers starts to fall, while low mortality rates increase the proportion of older dependents. This is the economic burden scenario. However, it is now recognized that a second demographic dividend is possible, again given the right conditions:[22]

> A population concentrated at older working ages and facing an extended period of retirement has a powerful incentive to accumulate assets—unless it is confident that its needs will be provided for by families or governments. Whether these additional assets are invested domestically or abroad, national income rises. In short, the first dividend yields a transitory bonus, and the second transforms that bonus into greater assets and sustainable development.[23]

As with the first dividend, institutional and financial structures need to be in place for this second dividend to occur. It is also being recognized that older workers can both boost their earnings, and thus their future assets, and contribute directly to the productivity of the economy through working longer. Indeed, there has been a general increase in the percentage of those over 50 who are now in the workplace in the advanced economies, and over one-third of this age group in the G7 countries (Canada, France, Germany, Italy, Japan, the UK, and the US), for example, recently reported their interest in working after retirement age. However, the education, training, and skills upgrading of this group will be essential. Indeed, lack of training across the life course and the subsequent low employability of older workers have been identified as major barriers to increasing the employment rate of older workers in OECD countries.[24] As I and colleagues have described elsewhere:

> The ageing population is driving society toward a more fluid interpretation of retirement. Historically, retirement has been viewed as a permanent exit from the labour force. That view may no longer be appropriate. Longer life spans provide more opportunity for workers to exit one occupation and enter another.... We may see workers exit, reconsider, and then re-educate in preparation for a major career change.... The experiences of older workers might modify our career models to include intense work periods followed by mini-retirements or sabbaticals; the sequence might be repeated several times over an individual's work life, and could involve multiple occupational changes.[25]

Increased productivity, increased savings, and—given the high level of wealth currently accumulated by older populations—continued consumption together with the ageing of populations may not herald the scenarios currently being forecast.

The challenge of increasing longevity

In terms of increasing longevity, the challenges could well become more demanding over the coming decades: obesity, antibiotic resistant bacteria, and increasing pressure on health service provision are all possible threats. However, things could well improve. As the US National Research Council pointed out, 'continued advances in biomedicine, especially a cure for cancer or Alzheimer's Disease could have remarkable effects, as would basic advances that slow the process of aging'.[26]

This aspect of the so-called grey burden is driven by falling mortality rates at older ages. This quote comes from the US, where in 2030 those aged 80 and over are projected to account for 5.4 per cent of the US population, up from 3.8 per cent in 2015.

Similarly, within the EU27, those aged 80 and over will almost equal the young, at around 12 per cent of the population, as this older group almost triples in size from 23.7 million in 2010 to reach 62.4 million in 2060. Such extreme ageing heralds a series of challenges for the provision of health and social care. Over the past 40 years, health care costs in most of the advanced economies have been rising on average at between 1 and 2 per cent faster than GDP.[27] The European Commission '2012 Ageing Report' gave a clear warning to member states:

> 75 per cent of the EU Member States spend between 11 to 15 per cent of their resources on health care. Growing public health care expenditure raises concerns about its long-term sustainability. Whilst public health expenditure in EU27 was at 5.9 per cent of GDP in 1990 and 7.2 per cent of GDP in 2010, the projections show that expenditure may grow to 8.5 per cent of GDP in 2060.[28]

Public spending on health care now accounts on average for 14.6 per cent of total government spending in the EU, ranging from 7.2 per cent in Cyprus to 18.8 per cent in Slovakia. In addition, while the share of public spending in the EU member states is increasing, private financing is also increasing as a proportion of total health care funding.

We can explore the impact of extreme population ageing on the provision of health care, and the degree to which ageing alone is contributing and will continue to contribute to the rising health care costs in the advanced economies. First, the age structure of a population is clearly an important determinant of health care costs. Costs are high for infant and maternal care and rise again as we age, from around age 55 for men and 60 for women. However, the largest proportion of health expenditure per person occurs in the final year of their life. Indeed, proximity to death is more important than age per se as a predictor of the consumption of health resources.[29] In many of the advanced economies, ageing of the large cohorts born in the middle of the twentieth century will increase the proportion of the population in close proximity to their death.

But there are other challenges as well. In particular, the total amount of ill health and disability is likely to increase, with accompanying pressure to increase health care spending. The type of ill health is likely to change from acute and infectious diseases to chronic conditions, and this will require major shifts in the allocation of health care resources and the configuration of medical and health care services. And importantly, the effect of decreasing numbers of younger people will reduce the number of people able to provide care.

As societies improve their population life expectancy, the total amount of ill health and disability in the population will rise because the proportion of the population with serious health problems will increase unless there is a significant improvement in the health of successive birth cohorts, which shows up as a decrease over time in age-specific prevalence rates. This has also been termed the 'epidemic of frailty',[30] as an increasing number of individuals surviving to experience the increased frailty and dependency associated with advanced old age. Therefore, if individuals do continue to experience increased frailty with age, then health care demand will increase as life expectancy increases. However, if there is a significant improvement in the health of successive birth cohorts, then it is possible that an increase in life expectancy will have no net effect on the prevalence of ill health and disability in the older population. This is because the proportion of the older population with serious health problems would remain unchanged, and thus any effect of population ageing on the amount of ill health in the general population would depend entirely on the increase in the relative size of the older population. In addition, while evidence suggests that per capita health spending does increase quite steeply once people reach their 60s, repeated analyses of age-related data on health spending have shown that proximity to death is more important than age per se as a predictor of the consumption of health resources.[31] In other words, health care spending is heavily concentrated in the last few years of life, so much so that some analysts have argued that ageing per se has virtually no effect on the way that the consumption of health care resources increases with age.[32]

But there will also be changes in the type of ill health arising from the shift from acute infectious disease to complex, chronic, long-term ill health and disability: the so-called *chronic disease burden*.[33] This will exert pressure for a major shift in the allocation of health care resources and the configuration of services. Whether because of population ageing or the rise in affluent life styles, it is clear that the rise in chronic disease will be driven in all modern societies by elements of both.[34] There is, therefore, a need in both the advanced and emerging economies to reallocate health and social care resources away from infectious and acute medicine towards preventing and managing late-life chronic disease. This will require the development and improvement of services for people with complex health needs, and this may require a large shift in the allocation of resources as well as large-scale organizational change.

The third factor concerns the impact of population ageing on a society's capacity both to provide workers to care for the older population and tax income to finance this. The changes in the dependency ratios, highlighted earlier, will particularly impact in the health care sector. In addition, demographic change will reduce informal family care through a reduction in the availability of younger family members to provide such care. This will increase the demand for formal care services at a time when the provision of overseas migrants providing health care is reduced as their own societies start to age. This issue is compounded because, as we have seen, the advanced economies are at the same time experiencing an increase in labour-intensive chronic disease care.

In addition, there are challenges facing all health systems in the advanced economies. For example, the large social inequalities in health status together with a set of non-demographic and behavioural factors such as the continually increasing range, sophistication and cost of health care interventions, the propensity of the patients to demand more health services, and our apparent willingness to spend more on health as we become more affluent will challenge even the strongest of economies.[35]

In conclusion, although a number of cross-national studies have considered the determinants of health care costs, only one has found that the age structure of the population, determined by the proportion of population aged 65 and over, is the explanatory factor.[36] Rather, it is the wider effects of income, lifestyle characteristics, and new technology alongside the effects of environmental factors which are driving up the demand for new advanced medical applications. Analysis of OECD data[37] reveals that in the advanced economies at least, per capita health care costs for those aged 65 years and over have increased at the same rate as for those aged less than 65 years. Furthermore, per capita spending on health care is reduced after age 85. This appears to be due to a number of factors: the lower demands made by these generations, a factor which may change as more demanding younger cohorts reach old-old age; the view held in many societies that, under resource constraints, spending should be directed to the young; and less research and thus understanding of advanced treatments for the very old.

Health care costs have thus increased far faster than population ageing would predict, and it is now widely accepted that techno-logical change in health care delivery has been the main driver, alongside increased demand from the population for expensive interventions and drug therapies. In addition, medical innovations now allow for the treatment of previously untreatable conditions, maintaining life but also increasing medical costs.[38] Up to half of the increase in health care spending in the advanced economies over the past 50 years appears to have come from the use of increas-ingly sophisticated medical technologies.[39]

Longer, healthy lives or just longer lives?

Another key question concerns the relationship between long lives and healthy lives. There have been several theories put forward to explain the interaction between life expectancy and disability. The *compression of morbidity* hypothesis[40] suggests that disability and frailty is compressed towards the end of life at a faster pace than death rates. Therefore, people are expected to live not only longer but also in better health. Alternatively the *expansion of morbidity* hypothesis[41] claims that the decline in mortality is largely due to the decreasing death rate from diseases rather than due to a reduc-tion in their incidence. As a result, falling mortality is accompanied by an increase in morbidity and disability. The *dynamic equilibrium* hypothesis[42] suggests a counterbalancing effect between the two: decreasing prevalence/incidence of chronic diseases and decreasing fatality rates from such diseases. This is leading to a longer prevalence of periods of living with disability towards the end of life.

There is now evidence from several countries which enable us to explore these ideas. The main evidence from the US is that chronic disability prevalence decreased in the US between 1982 and 2004. Younger cohorts of older persons are living longer and in better health, and there is good evidence of a compression of disability.[43] However, in Japan the gains in life expectancy prior to 1995 were mostly in years of good self-rated health, while the gains thereafter were in years of poor self-rated health. The data here suggest that life expectancy has been increasing faster than healthy life expectancy since 1995.[44] Similarly, in Singapore between 1995 and 2005, the proportion of life expectancy without mobility limitations declined at all ages and for both genders, with women still experiencing a higher proportion with mobility problems compared to men.[45] However, in Germany between 1984 and 2003, life expectancy without severe disability increased faster than life expectancy.[46]

A key study in the UK[47] explored three scenarios for the changing relationship between life expectancy at age 65 and disability-free life expectancy at age 65 between 2006 and 2026 (Figure 17). The first scenario looked at the UK ageing population per se; the second considered worsening health; and the third assessed the impact of improving health. When considering the portion of remaining life expectancy at age 65 that is disability free, it appears that while the years in good health increase, the years which are free from disability as a percentage of remaining life decrease in all three scenarios. In other words, while we may be increasing both years of life and years of healthy, disability-free life, as a percentage of life post-age 65 we are slightly increasing the years with disabil-

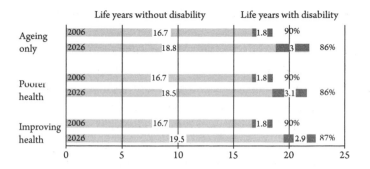

FIG 17 Life expectancy and disability-free life expectancy

ity. So taking the current ageing population as it is, by 2026 we would have seen an increase from 16.7 to 18.8 years disability free — that is from age 81.7 to 83.8 on average without disability—but we would have seen our years beyond that with disabilities increase from 1.8 to 3 years. If the UK population's health was to be reduced, then we would see an increase to 18.5 years disability free—that is from age 81.7 to 83.5 on average without disability—but our years beyond that with disabilities would increase from 1.8 to 3.1. If on the other hand our population health was to improve, then we would reach 19.5 years post-age 65 without disabilities by 2060, but the number of disabled years beyond age 84.5 would increase to 2.9 before we died. In all cases, this represents a slight increase in the percentage of time we spend with disabilities. What is clear, however, is that some disabilities (e.g. dementia and musculoskeletal diseases) will increase while others (e.g. cardiovascular and chronic respiratory diseases) will decrease.

Here lies what is possibly the greatest challenge. Epidemiological evidence suggests that the onset of disability is pushed back into later ages. Conditions which were prevalent within the 60 and 70 year age groups are now being delayed in some populations until the 70s and 80s respectively. A 70-year-old European now has the probability of dying today comparable to that of a 57-year-old some 50 years ago. This is primarily the effect of healthy living and tackling disease. But will these gains in both the number of healthy years and the total number of years of life continue as we increasingly turn to science and technology to extend our lives? Or will the increasingly scientific and medical drivers of longevity increase our life expectancy only for us to live for longer and longer with disease, disabilities, and frailties?

CHAPTER FOUR

Youth: Peril or Dividend?

Twenty-first century international security will depend less on how many people inhabit the world than on how the global population is composed and distributed.[1]

From continent to continent and across race and religion, the 'demographic' of insurgency, ethnic conflict, terrorism, and state-sponsored violence holds constant. The vast majority of recruits are young men, most of them out of school and out of work. It is a formula that hardly varies, whether in the scattered hideouts of Al Qaeda, on the backstreets of Baghdad or Port-au-Prince, or in the rugged mountains of Macedonia, Chechnya, Afghanistan, or eastern Colombia.[2]

This second quote starts a 2012 paper written by a member of the US Department of Defence.[3] It continues: 'one thing is certain—the demographics of Egypt and throughout the region have played an important role in the widespread instability. With this in mind, communities, countries, regional organizations, and the international community must enact, monitor, and assess policies that provide youth with "decent work" and social engagement in order to avert future crises.' Not only here but in numerous other papers written in the aftermath of the Tunisian and Egyptian uprisings of 2012, the 'youth bulge' was heralded as one of the major factors behind the so-called 'Arab Spring'.[4]

The youth bulge is conventionally defined as large cohorts between the ages of 15 and 24, expressed as a percentage of the total population. It is widely acknowledged that when the main factors leading to political instability—poverty, urbanization, and unemployment—intersect with a large youth bulge, the chances of conflict are increased. Currently, half the world's population is under age 25, with some 1.2 billion aged between 15 and 24. This is the largest youth cohort ever to transition into adulthood. Youth represents one-quarter of the global working-age population, but accounts for 40 per cent of total world unemployment. Members of this age group are three times more likely to be unemployed than other workers,[5] and it is claimed that young people make up almost 60 per cent of the global poor[6]—though this is also likely to include children. The large size of the cohort increases competition for limited jobs and other opportunities,[7] and as rural employment declines and urban manufacturing and service occupations increase, many young people find themselves migrating to large cities in search of work:

> Without the right policy environment, countries will be too slow to adapt to their changing age structure and, at best, will miss an opportunity to secure high growth. At worst, where an increase in the working-age population is not matched by increased job opportunities, they will face costly penalties, such as rising unemployment and perhaps also higher crime rates and political instability.[8]

For while a large number of young people can drive productivity if the economic structures and institutions are in place, if population growth exceeds economic growth or occurs at a time when countries are still in the early stages of economic development, such bulges can lead to high youth unemployment and poverty. Unemployment leads to feelings of alienation and increases availability for recruitment to political and criminal activities, and it is claimed that poverty plays a bigger role in political instability than ethnic diversity under these conditions.[9] It is now argued that it is the combination of large numbers of young men, particularly displaced ones, combined with high youth unemployment and subsequent poverty, which leads directly to civil unrest.[10] Indeed, it is suggested that as little as a 1 per cent increase in youth within a country results in a 4 per cent increase in the likelihood of conflict, and that in countries where the youth bulge makes up more than one-third of the population, the risk of armed conflict is 150 per cent higher than in the advanced economies with older age structures.[11]

However, it is also true that it is possible to have extreme youth bulges without unrest and civil strife. Indeed, unlike the MENA region, South East Asia, which has very similar demographics, was able to harness its youth bulge and convert it into the successful economic growth of the Asian Tigers: South Korea, Taiwan, Hong Kong, and Singapore. Similarly, China capitalized on its massive youth cohort, and now there are indications that the youth bulges in the Tiger Cub countries of Indonesia, Malaysia, the Philippines, and Thailand will replicate the success of the Asian Tigers. Let us look at the situation of the current youth bulge in the MENA countries and compare this with the Asian miracle, which emerged from similar demographics.

MENA countries

The MENA region has one of the largest youth groupings in the world. Around two-thirds of the population is in the age group 15–29.[12] Over the next two decades, huge youth populations will emerge in countries such as Iraq, Yemen, and the Palestinian Territories. Driven by high levels of fertility, currently these countries have over 40 per cent of their populations under age 15. The number of youth in Iraq is projected to increase by nearly 3 million—from 5.8 million in 2005 to 8.6 million in 2025; Palestinian youth will increase from 0.7 million to 1.3 million—more than an 80 per cent increase—and Yemen will see an increase of almost 70 per cent. Overall, the MENA region will experience an increase in youth to reach 100 million by 2035.[13]

While such a youth bulge presents opportunities for growth and prosperity, it has been argued that long-term prosperity and stability hinges on the opportunities afforded to these cohorts. Yet the youth in this region faces a variety of challenges: up to 40 per cent youth unemployment, lack of education, soaring house prices, delayed marriage, and youth dependency on families. It is further argued that the roots of youth economic exclusion are found in the formal and informal institutions that govern the education, employment, marriage, and housing markets. As a consequence, MENA men now have the highest ages of marriage in the developing world. In addition, unemployment and high housing costs, including poor access to mortgages and high rental costs, mean that these men are also delaying family formation. Credit to purchase independent housing is often limited, nor do they have the resources for a dowry, so young men cannot marry and set up an independent home, thus linking them into the relative stability of domestic responsibilities, including children.[14] It is this exclusion from stable adult life that is also key to the youth problem.[15]

Unemployment

Persistent and sticky unemployment has become the most significant economic and political issue faced by leaders across large regions of the world, from Europe to Central Asia, and the Middle East and North Africa. At the global level, unemployment is a manifestation of structural challenges: there is an increasing gap between education, skills and jobs; the global population is rising and we are witnessing increased protectionism; economic growth is out of balance at the global level, while policy-makers are urgently seeking plans to re-balance economies at the national level. These factors are impairing growth and hence job creation.[16]

Estimates suggest that youth unemployment rates are more than 40 per cent in Algeria, and that three-quarters of all unemployed in Syria and over 85 per cent in Egypt are youth.[17] Yet it is convincingly argued that the youth population bulge is not 'the' single or even 'a' major factor in explaining current levels of youth unemployment.[18] Indeed, the youth share of the working-age population was higher 40 years ago than it is today in most developing countries, including North Africa, where the youth bulge has been a focus of attention. While the demography of youth labour markets are important, it is naive to think that declining youth bulges will alone solve the challenge of youth unemployment. While the youth bulge was heralded as one of the major factors behind the Arab Spring,[19] the youth bulge in North Africa had actually peaked at 20 per cent between 1980–90 and has fallen since.

Instead, the key broad factors that have been identified behind the very high levels of youth unemployment are labour force growth, institutional and governance structures, economic and financial contexts, and education and skills. In the first decade of the twenty-first century, MENA's labour force—those either in economic employment or searching for such employment—grew at an average annual rate of 2.7 per cent, faster than any other region bar Africa.[20] The total labour force increased by 40 per cent and is predicted to increase by a further 80 per cent between 2000 and 2020.[21] The MENA countries are thus experiencing extreme labour supply pressures. Additional pressures are coming from the growing participation of women in the labour force. Driven by increasing educational participation and later marriage age, female labour force participation in MENA rose from 18 per cent in 1990 to 22 per cent in 2013.[22] It has been estimated that just to absorb these new entrants into its labour markets and reduce unemployment to an acceptable level, up to 80 million new jobs must be created.[23]

This is difficult to achieve, however, in the light of the other concerns, in particular weak institutional structures and governance, and the financial and economic contexts. Good governance is important to attract domestic and foreign investments into local economies to create employment and stimulate growth.[24] It needs strong legal systems both to reassure investors and to reduce corruption; economic policies which provide access to credit and protect property and assets to encourage saving and investment; trade policies to enable local products to have access to international markets; and basic transport and communication infrastructures to support both the purchasing of raw material and the marketing of finished goods. Yet it is generally recognized that by contemporary world standards both the rule of law and government transparency is weak in the region. This is seen as being responsible for the low levels of educational, fiscal, regulatory, and administrative reforms that would enhance the competitiveness of their economies, draw in capital, and increase employment opportunities.[25] In addition, MENA remains one of the least integrated regions in the world, having failed to take advantage of the expansion of world trade and foreign direct investment,[26] and some argue that it is the underdeveloped and underserving financial markets which have held back the region from realizing its potential growth.[27]

In recent decades, there has been a strong emphasis on the public sector as a source of employment. Around one-quarter of all employment in Tunisia and one-third in Jordan and Egypt is in the public sector, reaching over 40 per cent in Jordan and 70 per cent in

Egypt of non-agricultural employment. This has distorted the labour market and diverted resources away from a potentially more dynamic private sector.[28] Of particular concern is the fact that the public sector is now in decline in many countries in the region, and the private sector is not increasing sufficiently fast to compensate. Furthermore, the private sector has been hesitant to hire young inexperienced workers, and the alternative informal sector has little social protection or possibility for career progression and enhancement.

Importantly, there is also an extreme mismatch in the skills required by a modern economy and the skills held by the burgeoning young labour force. Employers, especially those in the modern employment sector, cite lack of suitable skills as a major constraint to hiring workers. The education system clearly does not provide youth with the skills they need for the modern labour market. The mismatch of skills and training in these labour markets is therefore a key factor; in particular, the education system has failed to provide the young with the skills demanded by the private sector. Some argue that it is these labour market mismatches which are at the heart of the high levels of unemployment in the region. In other words, the inability of the economy to create highly skilled work is matched by the inappropriate content and delivery of the region's education. Indeed, it is those with secondary, further, and tertiary education who have the highest rates of unemployment:

> On the eve of the Arab Spring in 2009, regional youth unemployment stood at nearly 24 per cent, the highest of any region in the world and almost twice the international average, a pattern that started and has persisted since the early 1990s.[29]

Unemployment among Egyptian college graduates is around ten times higher than those who did not go to college. Several commentators have implicated the concentration of unemployment among college-educated youth as a key factor in the 2012 Egyptian Revolution,[30] arguing that college-educated young men with high expectations are more likely to become radicalized.[31]

Arab Spring or Asian Tiger?

A large youth bulge need not, however, lead to civil unrest, unemployment, and poverty. The so-called Asian Tigers achieved their very high rates of economic growth during a time when they too had high youth bulges. Furthermore, demographically the greatest youth bulge had passed in both Egypt and Tunisia. Indeed, Tunisia had experienced its highest youth bulge some 40 years earlier, between 1975 and 1985. This is of particular interest, as Tunisia's youth bulge coincided with that of Hong Kong, with dramatically different outcomes. Hong Kong is part of the so-called success of the Asian Tigers—the high rates of economic growth experienced by Hong Kong, Singapore, South Korea, and Taiwan in the 1960s and 1970s. It is argued that this growth was propelled by the 'demographic dividend', that is, the rapid economic growth supported by changes in the age structure of a country's population as it transitions from high to low birth and death rates.

'A dream of Manhattan arising from the South China Sea' is travel writer Pico Iyer's much paraphrased description of Hong Kong. With an efficient and prosperous manufacturing economy leading to rapid economic growth, by 1980 Hong Kong had a per capita economy equal to southern European economies, and was second only to Japan in Asia. Yet Hong Kong and Tunisia both had large youth bulges between 1975 and 1985. As we saw earlier, the youth bulge in both North Africa and South East Asia peaked at 20 per cent between 1980 and 1990, and has fallen in both cases since. Hong Kong reached its highest percentage of 15–24 year olds in 1975 at nearly 25 per cent, falling to 22 per cent and then 19 per cent over the next decade. Tunisia reached its highest youth bulge at the same time—with 21 per cent of its population aged 15–24 during this decade. Similarly, Hong Kong's working population peaked at 70 per cent in 2005 and 2010, and Tunisia's at 67 per cent in 2010. Yet during its most vulnerable time for youth issues—1975–85—Hong Kong was experiencing considerable growth, and has continued to do so. By contrast, Tunisia has continued to stagnate, even now when it has its highest ever percentage of workers.

So there must be other things going on—and these focus around health, education, and governance. In Hong Kong, there were low levels of taxation and subsidized public housing, which had consequences for wage rates, along with government intervention to create a social infrastructure, which assisted Hong Kong entrepreneurs to respond to the rapidly changing global economy. There was a flexible labour market allowing the shift from manufacturing textiles to technology, and then to a financial centre accompanied by public expenditure on health, education, and social welfare, and public/private investment in infrastructure, with an emphasis on housing and transport including sea and air ports, roads, and bridges. These all contributed to Hong Kong's success.[32]

Demographically, however, we should note one thing. It has long been argued that the 'demographic bonus' only follows 15 to 25 years after the onset of the fertility decline, and the striking difference between Hong Kong and Tunisia is that while Hong Kong was well into the fertility transition in the late 1970s, with a TFR already between 2.3 and 1.7, Tunisia's childbearing remained high—with TFRs between 5.7 and 4.9 at that time. Thus Tunisia was still constrained by a large proportion of dependent children. Currently, the TFR in Hong Kong is just above 1, while in Tunisia it has fallen to 2. It is also interesting to compare the two regions in this aspect. The youth bulge in both North Africa and South East Asia peaked at 20 per cent between 1980 and 1990. At that time, the TFR of South East Asia was between 3 and 4, while it was between 5 and 6 in North Africa. It currently stands at 2.23 for the South East Asian region and 3 for the North African region.

Youth bulge into demographic dividend

The question is: how can governments ensure that youth bulges contribute to demographic dividends and not to civil unrest? This is what we turn to now—the potential of the demographic dividend.

There has been a long debate around the relationship between population and economic growth. On the one hand, it is argued that rapid growth in population size is negative for economic development, while on the other hand the view is that such population growth can lead to expanding markets and encourage economic growth, which in turn allows the development of public benefits such as education and health. It is, however, recognized that it is population structure which is of more importance than population size per se. As a country's TFR falls, child dependents (those aged under 15) begin to decrease relative to the adult working-age population aged 15 to 64. This usually occurs late in the demographic transition when a series of large birth cohorts are followed by a set of far smaller ones as birth rates fall. Families are thus able to concentrate their resources on the education, health, and well-being of fewer children, who as a consequence have a higher chance of survival. In addition, women with fewer children to bear and raise are able to enter and contribute to the formal labour market. For a short period of time, countries will need to spend less on education and other child-related benefits, and can capitalize on the increased productivity and savings from its large proportion of workers.

There is therefore a shift in the allocation of both individual and societal resources from investing in children to investing in physical capital, health, education, other public goods, and technological progress.[33]

It also increases the potential for high savings rates, particularly as the consumption needs of large numbers of dependent children are reduced. With fewer people to support, a country can take advantage of greater per capita output and economic growth, thereby producing the demographic dividend. While the youth dependency ratio continues to decrease or remain low, the potential dividend exists. In addition, this allows society to increase its aggregate per capita income level, before the time the population becomes mature, and to accumulate assets which can be drawn upon to help finance the consumption needs of an older population. This will be necessary because eventually older dependents begin to represent an increasingly larger proportion of the total population, heralding the end of the first demographic dividend.

A demographic dividend may thus be defined as the tendency for economic growth to be spurred by rapid growth of the working-age share of the population.[34] It should be stressed, however, that the dependency ratio is not just the ratio of the non-working-age to working-age population, but the ratio of actual non-workers to actual workers. The difference between the two is determined by the extent of absorption into work of the available labour force, which takes account of both underemployment and unemployment.[35]

The two main factors are thus demographic in terms of fertility reduction, and economic in terms of increased productivity and savings. But of most importance here is the fall in TFRs, as this means that the working-age population is not constrained by large numbers of dependent children; women are released for economic activity; and the production and consumption of young workers, unhindered by large numbers of child dependents, can drive the economy. As we saw, the economic, governance, and institutional context needs to be advantageous as well. Good economic management, with efficient financial and labour markets, supported through strong governance and institutional structures, is essential. There must be flexibility in the labour market to allow expansion and policies to encourage investment, and a skilled working population which is benefiting from good-quality health and education systems. These are required to enable the demographic dividend. Economic growth is thus not necessarily an outcome of increases in the working-age population.

In summary, we can say that demographic dividends are a composite of five distinct drivers: an increase in those of working age; a diversion of resources from young dependents to investment in human and physical capital; an increase in female economic activ-

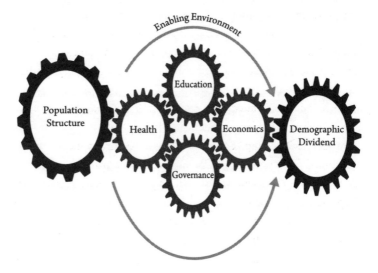

FIG 18 Policies facilitating a demographic dividend

ity following a fall in childbearing; an accumulation of capital by the working population to invest in the economy; and incentives to save with the realization of longevity and an extended period of late-life non-economic activity. As illustrated in Figure 18, key institutional frameworks in respect of education, health, governance, and the economy must be in place.

Many Asian countries will experience the opportunities of the demographic dividend over the next few decades. Demographically, China's and Thailand's demographic dividend period is forecast to last until 2035–40, Malaysia until 2045, and India and Indonesia until 2050.

First there was China, now there is India

The situation of China and India is of particular interest because there is a clear demographic relationship between China's demographic dividend and the lag in India's, which may be directly related to the difference in childbearing rate. Until the 1950s, the childbearing rates of both countries were similar, as was their economic growth, despite very different political systems. Both countries commenced a system of controlling population growth through restricting births, but while China's continued, culminating with the successful one-child policy from 1981, India's faltered. As a result, fertility fell and GDP grew in China, while India lagged behind as its dependent child population grew. Between 1980 and 2000, China's demographic dividend accounted for 15 per cent of China's economic growth based on the growth of the actual workforce and not the labour force. Of particular importance was the role of rural–urban migration, which allowed the young labour pool to move from economically declining rural areas to economically growing urban ones.

However, now that India's TFR is falling—especially among the burgeoning middle classes—there is also a debate about whether,

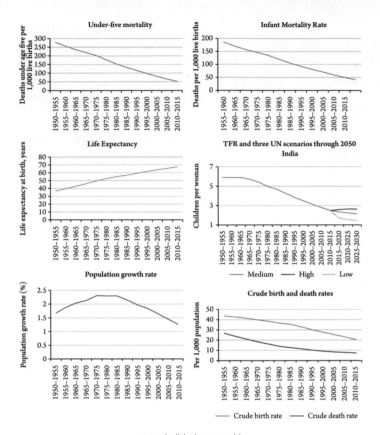

FIG 19 India's demographics

and if so when, India will overtake China as the major global economy. India's population is deemed to have reached 1.25 billion people, currently with a TFR of 2.5 and live expectancy at birth of 66 years (Figure 19). There is, however, considerable variation between states and between urban and rural areas, as Table 5 illustrates for TFRs. The economic growth is focused in the rapidly expanding urban areas, home to the growing population of middle

	Total	Rural	Urban
Andhra Pradesh	1.8	1.9	1.6
Assam	2.5	2.7	1.6
Bihar	3.7	3.8	2.7
Chattisgarh	2.8	3.0	1.9
Delhi	1.9	2.1	1.9
Gujarat	2.5	2.7	2.1
Haryana	2.3	2.5	2.0
Himachal Pradesh	1.8	1.9	1.3
Jammu and Kashmir	2.0	2.2	1.4
Jharkhand	3.0	3.2	2.1
Karnataka	2.0	2.1	1.7
Kerala	1.8	1.8	1.8
Madhya Pradesh	3.2	3.5	2.2
Maharashtra	1.9	2.0	1.7
Odisha (Orissa)	2.3	2.4	1.6
Punjab	1.8	1.8	1.7
Rajasthan	3.1	3.3	2.4
Tamil Nadu	1.7	1.8	1.6
Uttar Pradesh	3.5	3.7	2.7
West Bengal	1.8	2.0	1.3
India	2.5	2.8	1.9

TABLE 5   TFR by rural/urban location for selected states, 2010

Data source: India, Registrar General (2012) *Sample Registration System: Statistical Report 2010.*
New Delhi: Vital Statistics Division, Office of the Registrar General as cited in Table 1, p. 164,
Pradhan, I. and Sekher, T. V. (2014) 'Single-Child Families in India: Levels, Trends and
Determinants.' *Asian Population Studies,* 10(2), 163–75.

class Indians, some 350 million of them, often alongside populations living in poverty and deprivation. Inequality is one of India's
biggest challenges.

Demographically, China's working population will begin to
decline from 2015, and in 2027 will fall below India's, which has
been growing steadily over the past few decades (Figures 20
and 21). China's total labour pool has reached 1 billion, set to fall

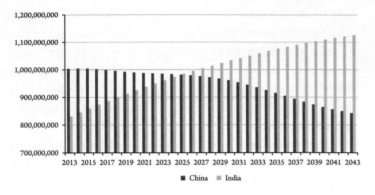
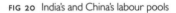

FIG 20 India's and China's labour pools

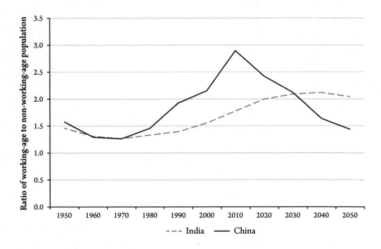

FIG 21 Growth of the working-age to non-working-age populations in India and China

back by about 68 million over the next two decades. India's will grow from about 800 million currently to reach just over 1 billion by about 2033. However, as we have discussed, just to have a large proportion of the country of working age does not guarantee the demographic dividend—and some argue that India does not have the stability, governance, and infrastructure to successfully capitalize on its demography.

One of the concerns is that the growth in employment required to accompany the rise in the numbers of workers will not occur in India. A second concern is the ability of India to boost its human capital through education and health programmes. For example, while the educational investment in India as a ratio of educational spending to GDP matches that in China (and indeed the public share in India is larger), the educational outcomes have diverged. It is thus argued that India faces a major deficit in the areas of education and health, which could adversely affect the conversion of a growing labour force into an effective workforce. In addition, if we take gender differences into account and again look not only at the available labour pool but at actual gender-specific participation rates, then due to the very much higher female participation rates in China compared to India, the shift in the demographic dividend bonus between the two countries also looks less likely.

What has happened elsewhere?

As is clear from Figure 22, there is shifting relationship across time in relative size of labour pool to the total population.

SOUTH KOREA

In 1950, just over half the population was of working age, with an extraordinary 42 per cent under age 15. South Korea prioritized access to family planning throughout the 1960s and 1970s through

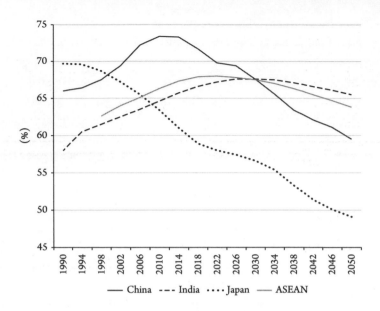

FIG 22 Labour pool as a percentage of total population, selected countries

a system of promotion by local health centres and home visits by care workers. As a result, the country's TFR dropped from 5.4 in 1950 to 2.9 in 1975, reaching a low of just over one child per woman in 2005. By 2010, the percentage of children had fallen to 16 per cent while those of working age had risen to nearly three-quarters of the population. Emphasis was also placed upon expanding health care facilities and encouraging health insurance, and by 2010 South Korea had one of the highest life expectancies in the world at 76.5 years for men and 83.2 for women. Education was also prioritized, with 99.2 per cent of all children in primary and secondary school.[36] However, over the next 20 years, South Korea's labour pool will shrink by some 11 per cent, and the cohort of young workers entering employment will fall by nearly one-third.

THE TIGER CUBS: INDONESIA, MALAYSIA, THE PHILIPPINES, AND THAILAND

Figures 23 to 25 illustrate the changing workforce in these four countries, alongside other selected Asian countries. The Philippines is set for considerable growth in its labour pool, with a 34 per cent increase over the next 20 years, with Malaysia and Indonesia at around 20 per cent growth. On the other hand, Thailand's labour pool is expected to shrink by around 12 per cent in that time. In addition, while the Philippines and Indonesia will experience a growth in the youth bulge, both Malaysia and Thailand will see the number of new entrants into the labour force fall.

Already the World Bank has warned the Tiger Cubs that they must improve public access to higher education and health care, develop ways to sustain productivity growth, contain health care costs, and expand the revenue base for social security.[37]

THAILAND

While not a member of the original Asian Tigers, Thailand is seen as a modern economic powerhouse of South East Asia. Like other South East Asian countries, Thailand prioritized health, education,

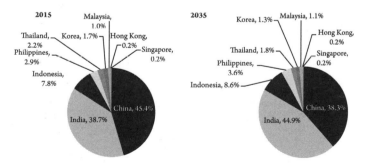

FIG 23 Change in the workforce in selected Asian countries

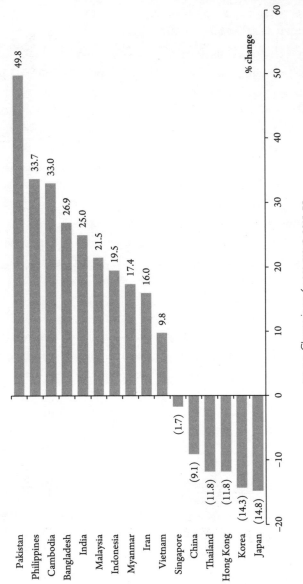

FIG 24 Change in 15–64 age group, 2015–35

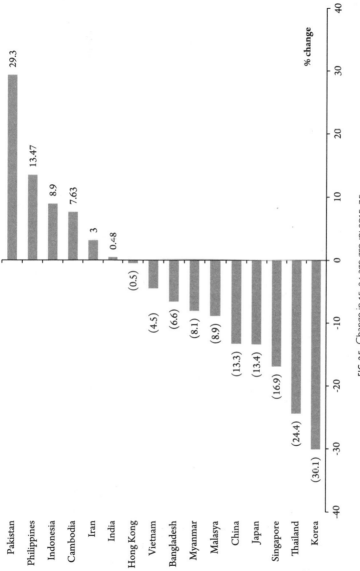

FIG 25 Change in 15–24 age group: 2015–35

and family planning as part of its overall development goals.[38] The result was a dramatic shift in its population age structure (Figure 26). In 1970, 52.4 per cent of the population was of working age, with 44.1 per cent under 15. Thailand's TFR dropped from 5.05 in 1970 to 2.30 in 1985–90, reaching a current rate of 1.49 children per woman in 2010. By 2010, the percentage of children had fallen to 19.3 while those of working age had risen to 71.8 per cent of the population. This is reflected in the changing relationship between labour income and consumption (Figure 27).

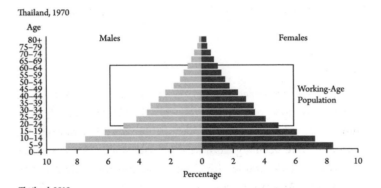

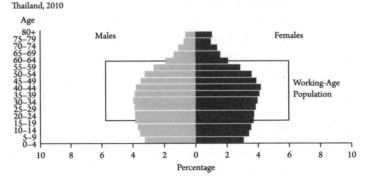

FIG 26 Thailand's demographic dividend

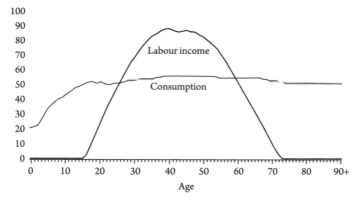

FIG 27 Life-cycle production and consumption of a Thai worker

VIETNAM

Though not recognized as one of the four Tiger Cubs, Vietnam is another country poised for a demographic dividend. Family planning efforts are carried out by both the public and private sectors, and they have been a government priority since the 1980s, when the National Committee for Population and Birth Control was established. As a result, Vietnam has seen a dramatic fall in its TFR, from 7.1 in the early 1970s to 1.9 in 2000, currently standing at around 1.7. In 1970, just over half (52 per cent) of the population was of working age, with 43 per cent under age 15. By 2010, the percentage of children had fallen to 24 per cent while those of working age had risen to 70 per cent of the population.

LATIN AMERICA

Most countries in Latin America began to experience significant mortality declines after 1950, which led to marked increases in life expectancies at birth for both men and women. In 1950, life expectancy at birth for males ranged from less than 40 years in Bolivia and Haiti to more than 60 years in Uruguay, Puerto Rico, Paraguay, and Argentina. However, mortality began to converge in the latter half of the twentieth century,[39] and by 2010 this range was from 60 years in Haiti to almost 80 in Costa Rica, Cuba, and Chile. The same was true for women, although the variance is declining for both genders. Fertility has also declined rapidly, and again converged. In 1950, levels had varied from 2.7 in Uruguay to 7.6 in the Dominican Republic, and by 2010 this variance was from 1.5 in Cuba to 3.8 in Guatemala. In the most populous countries of the region, the declines have been from 6.1 to just 1.8 in Brazil, and from 6.7 to just 2.2 in Mexico. Interestingly, the fertility fall in the region has revealed some differences from the European model, which was also prevalent in Asia, in that unwed births and cohabitation have preceded the delayed union formation and parenthood found elsewhere.[40]

The age structure, while an important component of economic growth, is not all important, as Latin America reveals. Latin America has had a very similar demographic transition to East and South East Asia, with TFRs at or around replacement and a steady growth in life expectancies. Yet Asia experienced a GDP per capita annual growth rate between 1975 and 1995 of 6.8 per cent. In Latin America over the same period the annual growth rate was less than 1 per cent. There is a general acknowledgement that the institutional structures and lack of rigorous directed policy was responsible. The political and economic framework, within which the demographic change was occurring, was one of weak governance, unstable policymaking, and lack of openness to world trade. In addition, Latin America's demographic window of economic opportunity arrived before it had established strong education systems and health care. Furthermore, many of its governments were corrupt, and repeated financial disasters reduced both the inclination and the capacity to save, which, as we have seen, is an important component in capitalizing on the dividend. However the economic performance in Latin America might have been even more dismal but for the region's large fertility decline.[41]

The role of demographic change

It is thus clear that age-structural shifts are important drivers of economic, social, and political change. The contrast between Latin America and Asia highlights this. The changing age structure in the regions has been estimated to account for 11 per cent of the gap between Latin America and East Asia. However, demographic interaction with the other factors increases this to 50 per cent.[42] Thus, Asian countries pursued direct policies which created new jobs to capitalize on the growing number of workers, while Latin American countries did not.

Let's take the case of the BRICS: Brazil, Russia, India, China, and South Africa. It was not only the tremendous political and economic change which spurred on their growth—it also involved the decline of Soviet economics, the opening up of borders and free trade, the commercial platform of the Internet, and the rapid growth of low-cost containerization enabling the rich resources of these countries to be transported across the globe at a very low cost. It was also the demographic change which was occurring in these countries at the time—a rapidly growing population of workers and consumers, and an internal middle class unfettered by large numbers of child dependents.

We can conclude by agreeing that 'while the demographic transition produces favourable conditions, it does not guarantee that an increased supply of workers will be gainfully employed. Nor does it ensure that those who wish to save will find themselves encouraged to do so. Neither can it provide institutions to reinforce health advantages or to create the educated population vital to an economy built around high-value-added activities.'[43]

This is, however, a key piece of the jigsaw which should not be ignored.

CHAPTER FIVE

Too Many Children?

'Lions On the Move: The Progress and Potential of African Economies', the 2010 Report from McKinsey,[1] declared that the stagnation of Africa had drawn to a close, and the Asian Tigers needed to watch out. It was a replication of the view of *The Economist*, which had moved from Hopeless Africa in 2001[2] to the Hopeful Continent by 2011.[3]

Indeed, Africa's economic performance since 2000 is widely acclaimed[4] and there is evidence that GDP is now rising in many countries—in particular Cameroon, Ethiopia, Niger, Swaziland, Ghana, Uganda, Senegal, Mali and, South Africa are seen to have made strong strides in this respect since the 1990s.[5] Yet there are fears that these growth rates have been encouraged by the increased demand for commodities from emerging economies, especially China, which may be transitory. In addition there is concern that this growth trajectory has not been translated into sustained reduction in extreme poverty. There is thus a need for the region to establish growth which is internally driven, equitable, and sustainable.

While the 2010 report did hesitate to ask whether Africa's surge was a one-time event or an economic turnaround, it concluded that resource-rich Africa—both natural and demographic—had benefited from governments' action to end civil conflict and enhance the business environment, with long-term growth being lifted by its internal demographic and social trends, in particular growing labour force, urbanization, and associated rise in middle class consumption. In 1980, 28 per cent of African's lived in cities, by 2012 this had risen to 40 per cent, equal to the proportion in China, and larger than India (Figure 28). These urbanites include a growing percentage with 'discretionary income'—that income which may be used to purchase goods other than the essential basics. Furthermore, by 2040 the labour force of Africa will have topped 1 billion, larger than India's, which itself will have overtaken China's during the previous decade (Figure 29). The 2010 report ends with a cautionary note, however: 'if Africa can provide its young population with the education and skills they need, this large workforce could account for a significant share of global consumption and production'. A cautionary note indeed, given the experience of the more economically advanced MENA countries, and the role that falling fertility has played in their potential demographic dividends. As we saw in Chapter 4, the

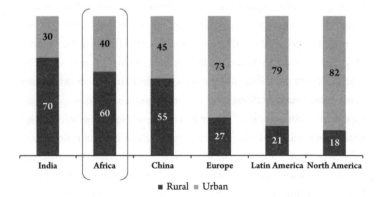

FIG 28 Share of the rural/urban population (%) by region, 2010

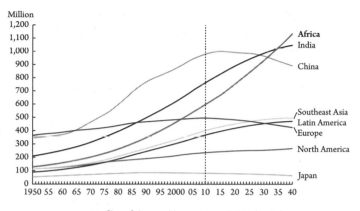

FIG 29 Size of the working-age population (15–64)

potential for economic growth arising from the emergence of Africa's large cohort of working age is significant, given the right conditions. The question for these countries therefore, is how to ensure the enablement of its demographic dividend.

A second key question, whether this apparent growth spurt in African economies has been translated into sustained poverty reduction, is also contested. What is more or less accepted is that without economic growth sustained poverty reduction across the continent is not achievable. Africa remains the world's poorest continent (Figure 30) and sub-Saharan Africa is one of the few regions of the world that has not substantially lowered poverty rates over the past 30 years. Various explanations are produced ranging from climate,[6] to corruption,[7] to civil conflict,[8] to continued population growth,[9] to poor institutions and poor infrastructure.[10] It is also argued that poverty is self-reinforcing—at the micro-level, poor households have no savings and no resilience against external shocks such as crop failure. When a large proportion of the country is engaged in hand to mouth subsistence activities, then the potential for economic growth is limited:[11]

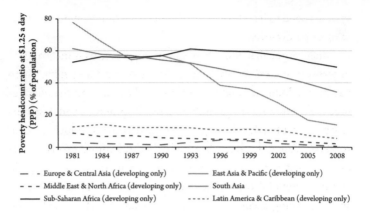

FIG 30 Trends in economic poverty by region

The connection between growth and poverty is self-evident; without growth a sustained reduction in poverty and wealth creation is not feasible. There is enough evidence to suppose that the growth narrative has changed, and the poverty numbers seem to be improving over time. The question remains would African countries be able to sustain these gains? What steps should be taken to prevent growth collapse and rise in poverty? Has the current growth episode been accompanied by sufficient momentum in job creation? These are the issues most policy makers and development partners ponder in contemporary Africa. Thus, the quest for 'inclusive' growth is now full steam in many countries.[12]

In particular the coexistence of a large traditional and informal sector with an emerging dynamic modern sector poses huge challenges for achieving a sustained reduction in poverty. There is also recognition that structural transformation is needed that addresses the role of the state, industrial policy, and trade;[13] the private economy needs to grow, foreign direct investment, or other sources of development finance need to be encouraged; and the health and education systems need to be reformed, including real commitment to innovation and new ideas.

Others argue that at the base of Africa's problems is inequality—in terms of income and wealth, in ethnicity, and in gender. There has been a long and highly contested debate around the effect of income inequality on growth and development, though generally it is accepted that the extensive levels of poverty which unequal societies can hold are a hindrance to economic growth.[14] Of new interest is the importance of gender inequality—in health, empowerment (also linked to education), and the labour market—and a growing recognition that this needs to be tackled. Even though this is one of the United Nations' Millennium Development Goals, progress has been limited,[15] especially in sub-Saharan Africa where seven out of the ten most gender-unequal countries in the world are to be found.[16] Women have less access to health care and education, both of which have an impact on their ability to successfully care for their own families'.[17] In addition, in most rural areas of sub-Saharan women and girls spend longer than men on time-consuming gender-defined activities such as drawing water, firewood collection, and accessing the rural markets.[18] For example, it is estimated that 40 billion 'women-hours' annually are spent on fetching water in sub-Saharan Africa.[19] And it is not only inequality in access to resources which is of concern, but also the need to enhance the ability of individuals to provide for themselves.

Releasing women from time-consuming tasks would enable them to contribute more effectively to the wider economy and well-being of families and communities.[20]

The two issues—sustained economic growth and poverty reduction—are clearly linked. While the economists and political scientists argue about the relative merits of their corners, let us look at the demographic case. The big question here is the relationship between high fertility and economic development.

A continent of child dependents

A large increase in the numbers of children puts a massive strain on countries that already struggle to provide enough schooling for their populations. Cities that are already bursting at the seams threaten to grow into increasingly unmanageable megacities, which makes it harder and harder for them to keep up with the demand for infrastructure and productive employment, and this in turn impairs their potential to act as engines of economic growth.[21]

As was discussed in Chapter 2, sub-Saharan Africa is not only the last region to initiate the fertility transition, it also has experienced a weaker pace of decline in fertility compared to other regions. While the global story on family size is generally very positive, with two-thirds of the world's countries now at or below replacement level—crudely defined as 2.1 children per woman of childbearing age, in sub-Saharan Africa women are still bearing over five children on average. This rises to over six or even seven in countries such as Chad, Mali, and Niger. This rapid population growth and high fertility threatens the well-being of individuals and communities across sub-Saharan Africa. As we saw in Chapter 2, the near 10 per cent projected increase in maximum global population this century largely arises from the fact that the fertility rate in Africa has declined more slowly than expected, and indeed appears to be stalling in several countries. Furthermore, even if the pace of fertility decline picks up, given the large young African population with current high levels of childbearing, the region faces many decades of rapid population growth and high child dependency. This not only has consequences for maximum world population, and the ability to feed that population, but also undermines the prospects for development and reduces the economic impact of the African demographic dividend. Most, though not all, governments in the region increasingly recognize that such high birth rates are reducing the potential for development, and African women are themselves calling for such measures which will improve their own well-being and those of their existing children.

The plight of Niger, the country with the highest childbearing rates in the world, illustrates this. Some 7.5 million Nigeriens, roughly half the country, are now without adequate food. Furthermore, the shrinking arable land beset by frequent drought is supporting a rapidly expanding population. Half the population—which is expected to grow from some 16 million today to 55 million in 2050, reaching 140 million by the end of the century—is under 15. Over one-quarter of girls are married by this age, rising to 60 per cent by age 19, and this is far higher in rural communities, where the majority are married at 12 or 13. Not surprisingly, similar proportions have given birth to children by these ages.

Slow fertility transition and fertility stalling

While the UN 2012 medium population growth scenario predicts that sub-Saharan Africa's childbearing rate will fall to around three children per woman by 2050 and come down to replacement later this century, some argue that Africa has different cultural and economic dynamics and that childbearing may well remain high. Sub-Saharan Africa is not only the last region to initiate fertility transition, it also has experienced a weaker pace of decline in fertility compared to other regions.[22] In addition, there is clear evidence of stalling in the rate of decline in childbearing (Figure 31). With the exception of the southern African countries, sub-Saharan fertility stalling seems to be far from exceptional:[23] the average pace of fertility decline slowed significantly in sub-Saharan African countries between the mid-1990s and the early 2000s. As many as two-thirds of the countries in the region experienced no significant decline in the first decade of the millennium, four have yet to start fertility decline, and ten have had fertility stalls (Table 6). Even in those countries where fertility *is* declining, the rate of decline is in most cases relatively slow.

There is currently a debate as to whether these stalls in Africa are but a minor pause in the course of the fertility decline, or whether this is an indication of deeper processes.

Achieving replacement-level fertility in Africa this century would bring huge benefits to African women, communities, and countries. If African women matched the replacement childbearing levels of other regions by the middle of the century, then sub-Saharan

Started fertility transition but now stalled	Pre-transitional TFR over 6	Started transition, stalled but now declining
Benin	Burundi	Ethiopia
Burkina Faso	Chad	Ghana
Cameroon	Mali	Kenya
Côte d'Ivoire	Niger	Madagascar
Gabon		Rwanda
Guinea		Senegal
Mozambique		Tanzania
Nigeria		Togo
Zambia		Uganda
Zimbabwe		

TABLE 6 Fertility transition and stalling

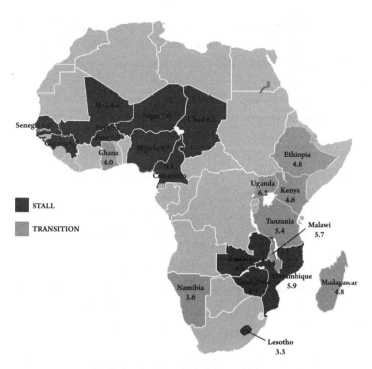

FIG 31 Family sizes in selected sub-Saharan African countries

Africa's population would stand at 1.76 billion by 2050, roughly 340 million fewer people than the UN's current growth scenario. Maintaining replacement until the end of the century from 2050 to 2100 would result in a population size of around 3.1 billion compared with the UN's current likely scenario of almost 4 billion. Indeed, a recent paper from the World Resources Institute, *Creating a Sustainable Food Future*, has called for fertility reduction as a means of tackling both the global carbon footprint and food security. Crucially, according to the World Resources Institute, a reduction in sub-Saharan Africa's population by the 340 million, which would arise if childbearing fell to replacement by 2050, would reduce global food demand by approximately 401 trillion calories per year, roughly 7 per cent of the predicted global calorie gap in 2050, and would reduce the growth in sub-Saharan's Africa's food demand by roughly one-third by 2050. Alternatively, if the regional reduction in childbearing was to stall and remain at its current level of 5.4, then sub-Saharan Africa's population will be approaching 3 billion by 2050 and over 16 billion by the end of the century.

It is now considered likely that the marked change of pace in fertility decline across sub-Saharan Africa may well be a regional trend. It is recognized here, as in other regions, that childbearing is reduced with higher levels of education, lower rates of infant mortality, and increased availability of modern contraception, all three also being associated with increased economic growth. Attention has thus been turned to understanding the *proximate determinants of fertility*. These are biological and behavioural factors which directly influence fertility, and through which social, economic, and other factors come to influence childbearing.[24] They include, for example, the likelihood of being married or in a formal union, breastfeeding, and use of contraception. These are factors which will vary between societies and cultures over time. In most societies, for example, childbearing happens within marriage, so a change in the age of marriage will affect fertility rates; similarly, different cultural norms and practices over the duration of breastfeeding or post-partum abstinence from sexual intercourse will have an impact on the likelihood of conception within marriage.[25] Some proximate determinants of fertility, such as reducing the time breastfeeding, may increase the likelihood of childbearing; others, such as delaying marriage, may decrease the likelihood of childbearing. And of course, both may be linked to the same underlying trend, such as increasing involvement of women in the formal labour market.[26]

Other factors may also be intervening that are specific to the sub-Saharan case, or to the specific circumstances within which Africa is now in transition, which may be different from earlier time periods. It has been argued, for example, that despite large differences in total fertility, there are strong similarities in the patterns of family building across sub-Saharan Africa, and that the persistence of high to medium-high fertility regimes across the region can be understood in relation to the wider institutional context in which African women's childbearing occurs:

> Historical institutions affecting attitudes towards childbearing, combined with contemporary social, political and economic uncertainty and institutional capriciousness, have inhibited the African fertility transition. Until these institutional dynamics, and their path-dependence are engaged with, Africa's fertility decline will remain slow.[27]

There is interest, for example, in the role of social security and long-term care programmes as a spur to household decisions around fertility reduction. A lack of such programmes may, for example, encourage women to continue childbearing to ensure their own old-age security. Fertility stalls or fertility reversals maybe a result of the deliberate reproductive strategies of couples. Because couples might have an economic advantage in producing children to be sent abroad later in migration, and who could remit money to the family, they may choose to have more children. In addition, possible reasons for the fertility decline to falter or stall also include the impact of the HIV/AIDS epidemic on mortality, poorly performing economies, the lower priority assigned to family planning programmes, and an apparent increase among some communities in the desire for large families.[28]

The position of Kenya illustrates this last point clearly. The number of children per women of childbearing age dropped dramatically in the last three decades of the twentieth century; falling from over eight children to five, the TFR then remained at just below five for the next decade, although there are indications that it may be falling again. Detailed analysis of the reasons for this suggests that the main factor was a shift towards women wanting more children. The evidence is clear that women with no education and Muslim women show dramatic reversals, while women with at least some secondary education have continued to want and have fewer births.[29]

It has been noted, for example, that despite wide variation in the TFR—from near replacement in South Africa to seven in Niger—there was a general increase in the intervals between births,[30] and it has been argued that postponement of childbearing in the region is a purposeful family strategy:[31]

> Parents cannot reliably trade child quality for child quantity, or predict that the foreign models of reproduction that now appear promising will not fall apart tomorrow. Prices for schooling, healthcare, or housing are extremely unstable, as are wages; even government employees are not paid reliably in some countries. Most employment opportunities are filled through social networks or kin relations, rather than according to formal skills or job experience; few people have access to formal credit. Buses do not run on schedule. Electricity and running water go out regularly, even in capital cities. In the rainy season, roads get washed out. Insect-borne diseases like malaria seem to strike more or less at random; the water-borne and sexually transmitted ones, from cholera to HIV/AIDS, only marginally less so. Mortality rates at all ages are high, and death often unpredictable.[32]

Postponement of childbearing, coupled with high levels of desired fertility, is described as a rational response to the uncertain personal and institutional context in which the majority of African women find themselves:

> Uncertainty about the future—property rights, education quality, employment prospects for one's children, and the absence of social welfare systems in most parts of the continent—militate against rapid declines in fertility.[33]

In other words, there is still a relatively high desired family size, though this has fallen over the past 50 years. Women still want children for cultural and economic reasons. Due to poverty and economic insecurity children are still required for labour, for late-life security, and increasingly for remittances. However, poverty and economic insecurity also means that there is uncertainty about health, education, jobs, food, and water—thus the best time to have the next child is unclear.

Children and adolescents: vulnerability

Even though there is awareness of the importance of investing in children in Africa, young people are among the poorest and most vulnerable individuals on the continent. Children are disproportionately affected by chronic poverty.[34] It is estimated that malnutrition and undernourishment is responsible for around one-third of child deaths and one-fifth of maternal deaths. As we discussed earlier, one-quarter of African children are 'stunted' in that due to extreme malnourishment their bodies and brains fail to develop properly—an irreversible condition affecting them for life. In some parts of the Sahel, for example Niger, half the children are stunted, and even in a country like Nigeria severely underweight children and stunting are found across the country (Figure 32).

In addition, there is a strong intergenerational transmission of poverty, which continues the cycle of deprivation as poor in utero

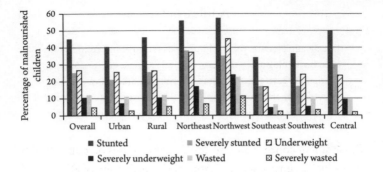

FIG 32 Prevalence of child malnutrition by residence, Nigeria

and child nutrition resulting from poor maternal and child health leads to long-term physical and mental stunting. Malnutrition and undernourishment impairs these children's immune systems, and prevents them from fulfilling their physical, intellectual, or economic, potential:

> Low levels of in utero and child nutrition resulting from poor maternal and child health lead to long term physical and mental stunting. Low levels of parental education and income serve to limit the potential for children's education and low parental income is also a key driver to early marriage and early childbirth, themselves determinants of higher than average maternal death and injury and lifelong resultant illness among girls and young women. Poor parents have poor children, and those children are more likely to grow up as poor adults because of the structural, social and health limitations faced as children.[35]

Of particular concern is the impact on young girls and how this is transmitted across their life course. Poverty leads to lack of schooling and early marriage, high fertility, and reduced well-being. There is now an increased interest in adolescent girls, and in particular those aged 10–14 in the transition from child to adolescent.

Adolescents

During adolescence, the world expands for boys and contracts for girls. Boys enjoy new privileges reserved for men; girls endure new restrictions reserved for women. Boys gain autonomy, mobility, opportunity, and power (including power over girls' sexual and reproductive lives); girls are systematically deprived of these assets.[36]

Government concern around adolescents focuses on public health issues such as unsafe sex facilitating the transmission of HIV/AIDS and other sexually transmitted diseases, early pregnancy with its associated high risks of maternal and infant mortality,[37] or the concerns raised in Chapter 4 associated with high levels of unemployment and civil unrest. It is, however, acknowledged that adolescent girls face a particular set of problems, as there is a risk of:

exploitative living arrangements; confinement to domestic roles and responsibilities; restricted mobility; inadequate and occasionally threatening school experience; unacknowledged work needs and compromising work situations; pressure to marry and begin childbearing early; and limited control over, and knowledge about, their reproductive health and fertility, even (perhaps especially) in the case of married girls.[38]

There is thus a need in these societies to create supportive institutional structures for pre-teen and teenage girls, enabling them to override the gender roles often imposed upon them by their families and communities to allow them to build the human capital required to function beyond marriage and motherhood. This is closely linked with the provision of educational and economic opportunities (Box 2).

However, as we observed earlier, many teenage girls are already wives and mothers, and need particular support to function in these roles at such young ages. Globally, over 100 million girls aged

> **BOX 2** Strategic priorities to empower the hardest-to-reach adolescent girls, particularly those aged 10–14
>
> ---
>
> - *Educate adolescent girls*: ensure adolescent girls have access to quality education and complete schooling, focusing on their transition from primary to post-primary education and training, including secondary education, and pathways between the formal and non-formal systems.
> - *Improve adolescent girls' health*: ensure adolescent girls' access to age-appropriate health and nutrition information and services, including life skills-based sexuality education, HIV prevention, and sexual and reproductive health.
> - *Keep adolescent girls free from violence*: prevent and protect girls from all forms of gender-based violence, abuse, and exploitation, and ensure that girls who experience violence receive prompt protection, services, and access to justice.
> - *Promote adolescent girl leaders*: ensure that adolescent girls gain essential economic and social skills and are supported by mentors and resources to participate in community life.
> - *Count adolescent girls*: work with partners to collect, analyse, and use data on adolescent girls to advocate for, develop, and monitor evidence-based policies and programmes that advance their well-being and realize their human rights.
>
> UN Joint Statement (ILO, UNESCO, UNFPA, UNICEF, UNIFEM, WHO)

between 10 and 19 have married over the past decade, making them vulnerable to the risk of young childbirth. Indeed, the WHO estimates that around 70,000 young girls die from the complications of pregnancy and childbirth every year. Girls who give birth aged under 20 have twice the risk, and those under 15 five times the risk, of dying in childbirth than women in their 20s. Indeed, pregnancy and childbirth are the leading cause of death for girls aged 15–19, with over 70,000 dying each year.[39]

The world's highest rates of child marriage (Figures 33 and 34) are seen in Niger (75 per cent) and Chad (72 per cent), and globally 4,000 girls under 15 are married each day:

> One of the gravest injustices suffered by young brides is the denial of education. The impacts of this injustice are multiple and far-reaching. Not only does it limit girls' earning potential, which increases the odds that they and their children will suffer from poverty, but it also reduces their odds of literacy and therefore their ability to take advantage of life-changing and life-saving information, including everything from agricultural techniques to sanitary practices. It also hinders the development of their confidence and voice, which leaves them with less access to decision-making over their own bodies and household spending. The knock-on ramifications of these deficits are huge, not only for their children—who are then themselves less likely to attend school and more likely to marry as children—but also for larger economies.[40]

Yet child marriage and its consequences are part of a large, complex network of household and family strategies and decisions.[41] In many countries where women cannot own their own land, marriage is the only way they can access land and thus food for themselves, and any future children they may bear. In Niger, for example, the ongoing food crisis has led UNICEF to express concern that more parents will use child marriage as a survival strategy, marrying daughters in return for dowries of much-needed animals and cash to feed their other family members. This will contribute to the high childbearing rate, which in turn is placing huge demand on the country's ability to feed itself. In other countries, where dowries are required, the higher price of older, more educated girls is seen to incentivize the family into early marriage. While in countries such as Uganda where high school fees pertain, young girls are

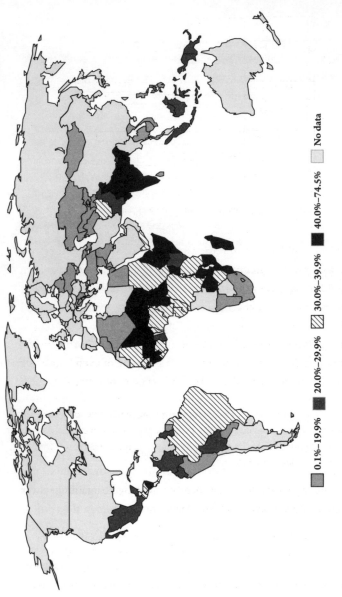

FIG 33　Prevalence of early marriage

0.1%–19.9%　　20.0%–29.9%　　30.0%–39.9%　　40.0%–74.5%　　No data

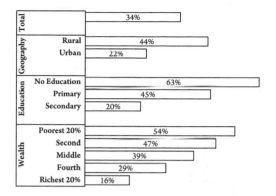

Total		34%
Geography	Rural	44%
	Urban	22%
Education	No Education	63%
	Primary	45%
	Secondary	20%
Wealth	Poorest 20%	54%
	Second	47%
	Middle	39%
	Fourth	29%
	Richest 20%	16%

FIG 34 Characteristics of child brides

promised to older men in return for these school fees. Other cultural norms define an unmarried state as shameful. In the Amhara state of Ethiopia, for example, which has the country's lowest education rate (with 60 per cent of adult women having never attended school) and highest child marriage rate (14 being the average age), marriage is seen as the only economic option for a girl. Furthermore, in Ethiopian Muslim communities it is shameful or even 'sinful' for girls to remain unmarried after they have begun menstruating:[42]

> When I was growing up I saw my mother struggling, unable to provide for us, and I was convinced by my peers that I needed a man who had money to provide. At the age of 12 years I got a man of 28 years who used to provide some basic needs.[43]

These young girls are driven by poverty and limited bargaining power into unequal relations which are ripe for abuse:

> Girls' age and lack of voice leaves them powerless to protect themselves over the course of their relationships as well. They are, for example, unable to insist on condom usage—dangerous as 'many men have gonorrhoea and syphilis, which they believe can be healed by having sex

with a young girl'. Given that older men often see children as a sign of their virility, girls are also prevented from using contraception.[44]

Potential for growth held back by dependents

It is argued that the growth in income per person could be substantial in Africa if countries were able to capitalize on the demographic dividend.[45] Achieving the UN medium fertility variant would boost per-capita income by 6.5 per cent in Nigeria to almost 27 per cent in Ethiopia by 2040 (Figure 35).

It is clear is that the large number of child and adolescent dependents in Africa is holding back growth and reducing the potential impact of the demographic dividend. The case of Kenya illustrates this. Over half the population is under 20, the dependency ratio is over 80 per cent—one of the highest in Africa—and around three-quarters of the population is still employed in the informal sector, primarily in small farms and informal urban activities. As is clear from Figure 36, expenditure on public goods and services is concentrated on the young who consume most of this through health and education. In addition there is also relatively high private

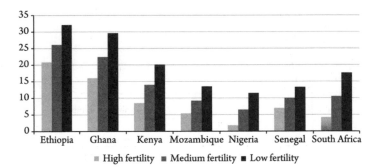

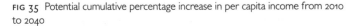

FIG 35 Potential cumulative percentage increase in per capita income from 2010 to 2040

education consumption among the under 20s, indicating further private transfers from working adults to younger dependents.

A similar picture emerges from Nigeria, as demonstrated in Figure 37, which shows large transfers to young dependents. While Nigeria has improved, still only around three-quarters of primary school-age children actually received formal education, and only half the population access health care services. Furthermore, the available tax revenue in Nigeria is low due to high unemployment and underemployment. Due to low taxation revenue relative to public need, the support for education and health programmes are dependent on consumption taxes on goods and other external sources, in particular from asset income—such as oil revenue—and foreign sources such as aid. Indeed, the high proportion of child dependents in relation to the working population means that human capital spending on health and education per child is low compared with outer countries. A lack of scholarships and bursaries means that households must find the cash to support their children's schooling; lack of health care reduces overall human capital and well-being.

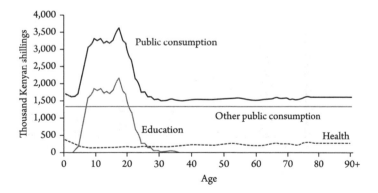

FIG 36 Per capita public consumption, Kenya 1994

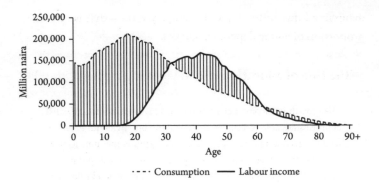

FIG 37 Age profiles of consumption and labour income: Nigeria, 2004

While Nigeria's economy has grown in the past decade, supported by strong government programmes to ensure economic growth and stability, these have had limited impact on poverty reduction. Many now acknowledge that Nigeria's rapid population growth and its continued very young age structure are holding back economic development and poverty alleviation. In particular, it is recognized that such public investments in early life health and education are essential for the future development of these countries (see Figure 37).

The challenge is thus two-fold—on the one hand the large number of child dependents is reducing the impact of Africa's potential demographic dividend, as the young working population has to transfer much of its income to young children rather than spend this on general consumption of goods which would help to drive the economy. In addition their investment in economic labour is reduced, in particular for women, as they are using much of their time and energy in caring for young child dependents. On the other hand, the large public investment in human capital development of the very young through health and education cannot be maintained due to the high dependency ratio—that is, the large proportion of young dependants to workers.

The role of education and developing human capital

The growth in income per person could be substantial in Africa if countries are able to achieve the demographic dividend. A rate of fertility decline that follows the United Nations medium fertility variant—the most likely future path—could boost per-person income by 6.5 per cent in Nigeria to almost 27 per cent in Ethiopia by 2040. Stronger investments in family planning and reproductive health programs could further accelerate fertility declines, leading to an even greater cumulative income boost and a larger dividend.[46]

The age structure of the least developed countries is clearly an ongoing cause for concern—one that can be tackled by a large investment in human capital development, in particular health and education. As we discussed in Chapter 2, there are three major drivers behind fertility fall—reducing infant mortality, increasing family planning programmes, and empowering women—and education has a positive impact on all three. Education not only empowers women, it also has a direct effect on the uptake of family planning technology, delays marriage and childbearing, and ultimately reduces the number of mouths to feed. Education lessens infant and maternal mortally, and empowers women to choose the family size they will bear.

There is a strong association between those countries with a high level of educated women, at least 60–80 per cent of the female population of reproductive age having completed at least junior secondary education, and those countries with below replacement fertility levels. Similarly, those countries with low female junior secondary education rates of below 40 per cent also have high

TFRs. A World Bank study, for example, found that for every four years of education that girls attain, fertility rates drop by roughly one birth.[47] Other research suggests that doubling the proportion of women with a secondary education reduced average fertility rates from 5.3 to 3.9 children per woman.[48]

In terms of empowerment, the effect of education on fertility is particularly strong in countries that still have relatively high overall childbearing levels.[49] Girls' secondary education is a tool for poverty alleviation, and results in social benefits to the whole society, equipping women with critical thinking capabilities and enabling civic participation and democratic change.[50] Research has also shown that while knowledge of modern family planning methods is now widespread, those women with high levels of education are more likely to adopt family planning methods than those with low levels of education.[51]

In summary, it is clear that there is strong association between those countries with a high level of educated women and those countries with below replacement fertility levels. Similarly, those countries with low female education have high levels of childbearing. A World Bank study, for example, found that for every four years of education that girls attain, fertility rates drop by roughly one birth. Another study found that doubling the proportion of women with a secondary education reduced average fertility rates from over five to under four.

There is also overwhelming evidence that education improves health and well-being, and reduces levels of infant mortality.[52] Girls and women not only face the challenges of high fertility and unwanted pregnancies; it is they within the community who are primarily responsible for infant and child health, immunization, and nutrition. Indeed, there is evidence that a mother's education is the most important determinant of child mortality, more important than household income or wealth, with each additional year of schooling being associated with a 5–10 per cent reduction in infant mortality.[53]

The evidence is clear that the enrolment of all African girls in secondary school education would have a significant impact on the numbers and timing of their childbirths, and result in a significant fall in childbearing in the region. Niger, for example, has one of the lowest educational rates in the world, with only 5 per cent enrolment in secondary school, less than 2 per cent of girls. Childbearing varies widely across the country, with the level of education ranging from four children per woman with secondary school education to over seven for those without education. In Ethiopia, with a far higher overall education rate, women without any formal education have on average six children, whereas those with secondary education have only two.

It is now accepted by most societies that education is a fundamental human right—one that all individuals are entitled to, regardless of their personal characteristics or circumstances. Yet it is a right which is beset by inequalities—between countries and between the genders. The Millennium Development Goals (MDGs) set the target of universal primary schooling by 2015. Yet there are still over 100 million children who are not in school and some 150 million more who are likely to drop out before they complete primary school. Over 60 nations—the majority in Africa—will be unable to ensure universal primary school education by that date.

There is further inequality between the genders, despite the fact that the MDGs also set the target of eliminating gender disparities in primary and secondary education by 2005, and of achieving gender equality by 2015. There is thus considerable variation in differential gender access to education at both the primary and secondary level. Indeed, half the girls in Africa will not complete a primary education. Worldwide, 90 per cent of primary school age children are enrolled in primary or secondary education, but only 77 per cent in sub-Saharan Africa. Sub-Saharan Africa does not only have lower educational attainment than other regions, it is also the region with the greatest gender disparity against women. The highest gender disparity in educational attainment exists in Benin, Burkina Faso, Chad, Malawi, and Senegal. In these countries, less than one-half as many women as men have completed any formal education. In 47 countries, girls are less likely than boys to enter the last grade of primary education. The most extreme situations are found in the Central African Republic, Chad, the Democratic Republic of the Congo, and Yemen, where girls have around two-thirds of the participation rate of boys. The region also has the lowest overall rate of participation in secondary education and the most severe gender disparities. In 2009, only 32 per cent of girls had any secondary school education, versus 41 per cent for boys. Only 27 per cent of pupils complete upper secondary school programmes, falling as low as 6 per cent in the Central African Republic, Niger, Somalia, and the United Republic of Tanzania. These inequalities persist because traditionally, in terms of educational opportunities, all societies have privileged males over females. Thus disparities in educational attainment and literacy rates today reflect patterns which have been shaped by the policies and practices of the past.[54]

A range of key barriers to universal education, and in particular universal secondary education, have been identified.[55] These include the inability of countries to meet the growing demand for education, both financially and in terms of trained teachers, and the inability of individual households to meet the direct and indirect costs of education (i.e. tuition fees, school uniforms, and time away from household chores or external employment). Estimates of how much it would cost to achieve both universal primary and secondary education range from $34 billion to $69 billion per year (with primary education being $6 billion to $35 billion per year and secondary education from $28 billion to $34 billion per year). There are considerable difficulties in producing accurate cost estimates, because of the uncertainties around estimating how to overcome the barriers, such as parents not enrolling their children in schools.

While there are concerns that Africa's childbearing regime is framed differently from other regions, the argument for expanding opportunities for and access to universal secondary education for all young people are strong.

CHAPTER SIX

Our Future Selves

The key challenge for both current and future societies is to maintain wellbeing across the life course, and within and between generations, as age structures change leading to significant implications for the redistribution of national and global resources.[1]

Summary

We started the book in Chapter 1 with life stories from women whose lives had been shaped by their demographic context. We have now explored the various dynamics influencing their lives and the significant age-structural shift which is occurring in most countries during their lifetimes. This is exemplified by South Korea in Figure 38. A Korean woman born in the same year as Samira, Varya, and Lisa, in 1975, will have moved from being a member of a large birth cohort at the base of the Korean population pyramid, to being a member of a large 70-year-old age cohort towards the top of the Korean population vase.

It is possible to make speculative predictions of the world in which our three women will live as 70 year olds in 2045, and indeed beyond—but they will be no more than speculative. We can, however,

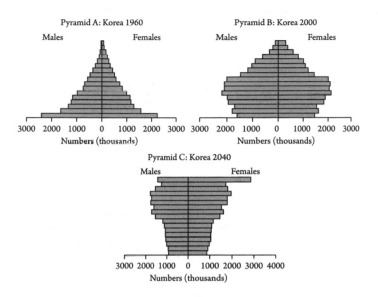

FIG 38 Projected age-structural change in South Korea 2000–40

identify certain trends which may influence our future world, and in particular we can project current demographic trends, supported by assumptions, which will provide us with a demographic framework for future societies. Figures 39, 40, and 41 illustrate the predicted age structure changes across the century—with a large fall in the percentage of children across the globe, and an increase in older adults. They also show where the workers of the world will live, moving from a concentration in Europe in 1900 across to the US in the mid-twentieth century, and then Asia dominating the scene until 2050, when Africa will have huge numbers of people of working age. We already know, however, that childbearing rates may not fall as assumed in sub-Saharan Africa, and that this region

a) 2000

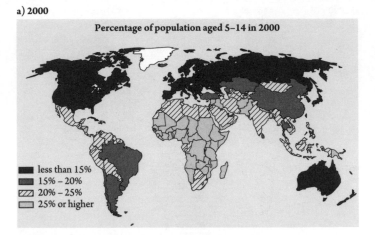

b) 2050

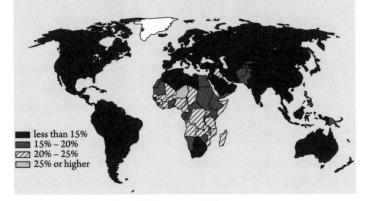

FIG 39 Map of children

a) 2000

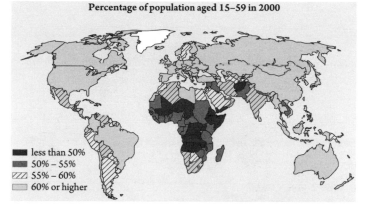

Percentage of population aged 15–59 in 2000

■ less than 50%
▨ 50% – 55%
▨ 55% – 60%
☐ 60% or higher

b) 2050

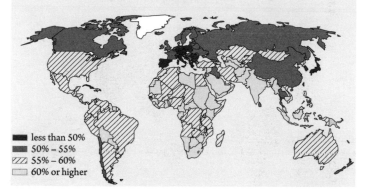

Percentage of population aged 15–59 in 2050

■ less than 50%
▨ 50% – 55%
▨ 55% – 60%
☐ 60% or higher

FIG 40 Map of workers

Percentage of population aged 60 + in 2050

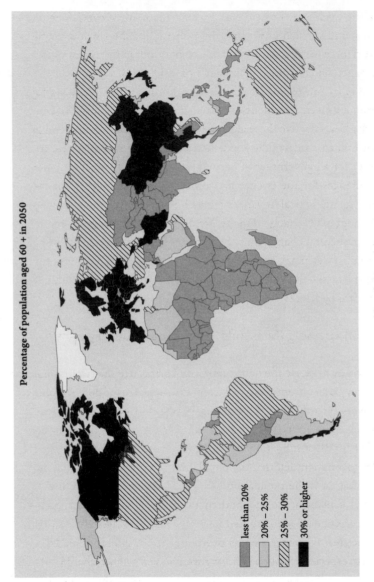

less than 20%

20% – 25%

25% – 30%

30% or higher

FIG 41 Map of older adults

of the world may be held back by huge numbers of child dependents, and we also know that the potential of the world's young workforce may be unreleased due to poor infrastructure and governance, and the growing influence of technology.

Let us now explore the preparation for this world. First, as governments introduce policies to change their age structure, we consider how effective these are and whether emphasis on promoting the human capital of the population should be the number one priority for all governments. Second, we highlight two other major challenges for the twenty-first century—environmental change and technological advances—and how they may interact with demographic change. Finally, we argue that the importance of age-structural change must be integrated into our understanding of human, societal, and economic development, and consider the broader issue that institutions developed for the twentieth century are dealing with twenty-first century challenges.

Addressing the trends through population policy

One way to tackle the demographic imbalances of the twenty-first century is for governments to attempt to manipulate the demographic drivers directly. In general terms, population policies are those which aim to modify the growth rate, composition, or distribution of a national or subnational population.[2] These might be introduced if a government felt that the population was growing or shrinking too fast, or if the population had an unbalanced age structure—with too many or too few children for example—or that its population was unevenly distributed across the nation to the detriment of some areas which were either overpopulated or underpopulated.

An explicit population policy is government action which explicitly aims at modifying a demographic outcome, such as the imposition of a cap on immigration, subsidized family planning services, or a direct ban on couples having more than one or two children. An implicit population policy is one which does not explicitly aim at modifying the population, but is understood to have a predictable demographic outcome. While few countries have direct population policies, many governments acknowledge that some of their policies have indirect demographic outcomes. A key example of this is the introduction of compulsory secondary education in the emerging economies and in the least developed economies, which, as we saw in Chapters 2 and 5, has had a positive impact on reducing high childbearing.

It is more or less universally accepted that reducing mortality rates within a population is a good outcome, and that most governments aim to do so through health policies. While currently there are no direct attempts to reduce the rapid decline in late-life mortality, if longevity continues to increase at current rates, leading to extreme extension of life, this may be an issue for public debate. However, here we shall focus on policies which directly or indirectly influence fertility and migration. In many of the advanced economies, governments are exploring policies to compensate for, or even to alter, the age composition of the population. These include encouraging changes in fertility and migration rates in order to increase the proportion of young people. In the emerging economies, including some in sub-Saharan Africa, governments have encouraged a reduction in fertility to slow population growth.

The modification of fertility trends

PRO-NATALIST POLICIES

Many European countries have adopted both direct and indirect pro-natalist policies deigned to raise the TFR and counter their age-structural change.[3] Most common is a general recognition that 'family-friendly' policies, aimed at supporting both children and parents, allow women to have the number of children they desire.[4] In most OECD countries this tends to be higher than actual achieved births.[5] These policies include affordable childcare, parental leave, housing subsidies, and other financial transfers and tax provisions, with some evidence that provision of childcare has the greatest effect.[6] Indeed, the fertility rate is highest in those European countries where family norms are flexible, mothers are active in the labour market, and childcare is well provided.

Thus, while some countries such as France have had clear direct pro-natalist polices for many years, others such as Norway and Sweden have family-friendly policies—such as flexible working and long, well-remunerated parental leave—which are seen to lead to large families. Others such as Poland, Italy, and Spain families receive payments for each child. Indeed, the UK explicitly states that it does not have a pro-natalist policy, and yet all British mothers, regardless of household income, until very recently received child benefit—payments on the birth of each child—which lasted until the child left school.

Romania pursued an active fertility promotion policy in the 1960s under the communist rule of Ceausescu, which used draconian measures to ensure large families with the explicit aim of raising the size of the Romanian population. Concerned about the low rate of population growth, and its consequences for industrial and military progress, the Romanian government introduced an explicit pro-natalist policy in 1966 which included a number of measures to increase the rate of childbearing. These restricted access to contraception, made abortion legally available only in certain limited circumstances, and increased allowances for large families. This had an immediate impact on fertility levels in Romania, and in the five years between 1965 and 1970 the TFR rose from 1.95 to over 3. This, however, was unsustainable, and when childbearing dropped back to 2.25 in the 1980s, the Romanian government imposed a strict abortion control regime, increasing the legal abortion age to 45 years or older, and only for women who had given birth to at least five children who were currently under her care. Despite all these measures, the TFR of Romania remained below 3, and following the repeal of the pro-natalist policy in 1989 by the new transitional government, the TFR fell and is now in line with other countries in Central and Eastern Europe at about 1.5.

France has long pursued an active, though less draconian, policy to encourage higher rates of childbearing. In 1939, the 'Code de la famille' was passed, introducing a series of pro-natalist policies. These included long periods of maternity leave, cash incentives to mothers who stayed at home to care for children, tax incentives, payments for third children, generous maternity grants, preferential treatment in the provision of mortgages and rental accommodation, and strong provision of childcare. Perhaps as a consequence, France now has the highest TFR in Europe at 2.1 children.

Sweden does not have an explicit population policy, but one which is recognized as leading to predictable demographic outcomes. The two-child family norm has remained strong in Sweden, with few one-child families and a stable level of childlessness. The country is seen to have *pro-cycle fertility*, in which childbearing goes up and down in relation to the country's economic business cycle. This appears related to Sweden's family policy goals of promoting good economic living conditions for all families and facilitating the combination of work and children for both women and men. This is achieved by the widespread provision of daycare centres and after-school services, parental insurance, and child allowance and other benefits. As a consequence, women remain in the labour market after childbirth, and both men and women take a period of parental leave after the child is born. In particular, this generous paid parental leave does seem to have facilitated increased childbearing.[7] Sweden is now introducing measures which will further enforce its aims. It has long been recognized that the very generous parental leave may disadvantage women in the labour market. Mothers typically choose to take longer parental leave than fathers, and this has been found to have a negative effect on women's careers and earning ability. In 2008, a 'gender equality bonus' was introduced to give an extra economic bonus to parents who share the leave more equally. Promoting shared responsibility for children, rather than allowing families to make the decision on non-economic grounds, has come in for some criticism. At 1.92 Sweden has one of the highest TFRs in Europe. However, even here it is clear that a complex set of factors influence decisions around childbearing, and policies designed to encourage increased childbearing have but a limited effect.[8]

Policies to reduce fertility

The first national family planning programme was launched in India in 1952, following the formation of the Family Planning Association of India in 1949. Programmes promoting family planning to reduce births began in many countries in Asia and Latin America in the 1960s in response to falling infant and child mortality rates and subsequent rapid growth in population. The number of developing countries with official policies to support family planning rose from only two in 1960 to 74 by 1975 and 115 by 1996.[9]

The potential impact of such policies is well illustrated by comparing the paths of Pakistan and Bangladesh. In 1971, when Bangladesh gained independence from Pakistan, the TFRs were similar at just under seven births per woman. But while Pakistan continued with its traditional family planning approach, Bangladesh adopted a new and active programme. Its successful community-based education approach, supported by provision of modern contraceptives, not only achieved a steady fall in infant and maternal mortality, but also a strong fall in TFRs, which halved to 3 in 20 years, and are now hovering around replacement level. Alternatively, Pakistan banned family planning in the 1980s, and by 1990 only 12 per cent of couples in the country used modern contraceptives. As shown in Table 7, Pakistani women have on average one child more than their Bangladeshi neighbours, and while it is assumed that Pakistan will also reach around replacement level before the middle of the century, the impact of delayed family programmes has had a significant impact on its child dependency ratio and its population growth. In 1970, Bangladesh had 7 million more people than Pakistan (59 and 66 million inhabitants respectively), but by 2050 Pakistan will have 107 million more (202 and 309 million respectively). Indeed, in terms of reducing childbearing, Bangladesh achieved through community education what India had achieved through a period of enforced family planning (Figure 42).

However, population policies have not always been successful, as has been seen in sub-Saharan Africa. The first countries to announce population policies in the region were Kenya in 1967 and Ghana in 1969. It took a further two decades before 30 further

	Bangladesh	Pakistan	India
1971	6.9	6.6	5.4
1981	6.2	6.5	4.6
1991	4.4	5.9	3.8
2001	3	4.3	3.1
2011	2.2	3.4	2.5

TABLE 7 TFR, Bangladesh compared with India and Pakistan

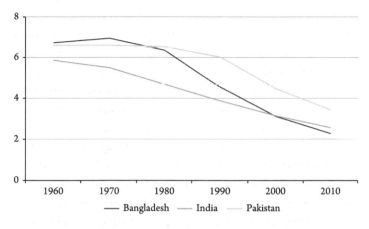

FIG 42 TFR, Bangladesh compared with India and Pakistan

countries adopted such policies, led by Nigeria, Senegal, and Liberia at the end of the 1980s. Programme adoption appears to have diffused across the region, adopted first in West Africa, then the Sahel and the south of the continent. Most Central and Eastern African countries did not adopt such policies. Even here, the motive for family planning policies does not seem to be driven entirely by a desire for population reduction. One explanation is that a set of traditional countries adopted family planning policies first, to illustrate their modern outlook, and then their neighbours following suit in order to gain legitimacy within the African community, and importantly with the global community in order to ensure the flow of foreign aid.[10]

Let us look at the case of Kenya. The first country in sub-Saharan Africa to adopt a policy to reduce population growth, it did not initially experience success. One decade later, it still had one of the highest TFRs in the world at eight births per woman, with a desired family size of seven children, and under 10 per cent of reproductive women using modern contraceptive methods. Concerted government efforts throughout the 1980s, involving widespread access to family planning supported by major information campaigns, nearly trebled contraceptive use, and the TFR dropped dramatically in the last three decades of the twentieth century, falling from over eight children to five. However, as we saw in Chapter 5, the TFR then remained at just below five for the next decade. But Kenya's new 2010 constitution places family planning within its fold: 'Every person has the right to the highest attainable standard of health, which includes the right to health care services, including reproductive health care.' A new national population policy is currently being developed with family planning at its core, and, in particular, the government will now cover the full cost of contraceptive commodities. The slow start, however, has allowed a strong demographic momentum, and Kenya's population, which had already quadrupled from 11 to 43 million in the 50 years since it started its family planning programme, is now predicted to reach some 97 million by 2050.

Ghana, the second sub-Saharan country to adopt a population policy in 1969 (revising this in 1994 to incorporate new and emerging issues such as HIV/AIDS, the environment, and gender) is a far more successful story. The adoption of a population policy in Ghana was in response to rapid population growth. The main aims were to increase the use of modern family planning methods, reduce maternal and infant mortality, and increase female secondary education rates—all being recognized as contributing to fertility decrease. While this has been successful in that the TFR has fallen from just under 7 in 1969 to under 4 currently, there is still wide variation, with an urban rate of 3.1 compared with the rural rate of almost 5, and those women with secondary education achieving 2.5 while remaining at 6 for those with no education.

Despite more than 50 per cent of the population now being urban, and a high level of female secondary education, modern contraceptive use is still low at below 20 per cent of the female childbearing population, a reflection of the still strong cultural and traditional beliefs and behaviours in the country. As a result, population growth rates are still over 2.5 per cent per year and the population has grown from 6.7 million in 1960 to its current size of 24.2 million, predicted to reach around 40 million by 2050. Still, this is only a threefold increase from the 1960s to now, compared with a fourfold increase for Kenya. In addition, Ghana will have a predicted sevenfold population increase in just under a century (1960–2050) compared with a ninefold increase for Kenya in the same time span.

One of the most famous population policies was China's one-child policy. This was a direct population policy aimed at reducing population growth through bringing down its TFR. A voluntary policy in 1978, which aimed to curb the population as it raced towards 1 billion, was followed by the instigation of the one-child policy in September 1980. A universal programme with exceptions for some ethnic minority groups and for those with a handicapped first child, it was implemented more effectively in the large cities in the east of the country than in the small agricultural communities of the rural west. Various methods of enforcement were used, ranging from widespread availability of contraceptives and close community and workplace monitoring, through preferential employment opportunities and financial incentives for those who complied, to the more extreme measures of forced sterilizations and abortions.

The policy was effective in the areas in which it was enforced, resulting in a steady fall in birth rates to below replacement by the mid-1990s. However, unintended consequences include a skewed ratio of men to women, as less-valued baby girls were removed through abortion, abandonment, and infanticide, and the existence of possibly millions of unrecorded second and third children, who face a life without formal education, health care, or employment. In addition, the age dependency ratios within China's population has been exacerbated, as long-lived parents and grandparents find themselves without a nexus of children to care for them within the family. Recently, couples where at least one parent was a one-child baby—the majority of young adults now—have been allowed to have two children. However, the indication is that most are choosing to stick to the one-child family model within which they themselves grew up.

Migration

Population movement—or migration—has the ability to transform population structures and sizes: within-country migration often leading to rapid urban growth and/or rural depopulation, for example. International migration often compensates for population decline or the need for young workers. While there are growing concerns in many of the emerging economies about rapid, and in places unsustainable, urban growth and the ageing and decline of the rural agricultural work force, our main interest here is on the long-term use of migration by the advanced economies to compensate for their ageing workforces, potential shortfalls in skills, and increased dependency ratios.

Immigration is thus seen by governments in advanced economies as having the potential to prevent population decline, maintain the size of the labour force and thus the support ratio, and slow the ageing of the population. Many governments, however, while wishing to attract or deter migrants, do not openly declare this to be a population policy. The UK, for example, does not have a population policy in terms of attempting to influence the overall size of the population or its age structure, nor does it openly declare a view on a desirable size or age composition. The UK does, however, have an immigration policy which states that 'immigration enriches our culture and strengthens our economy and therefore we want to attract people to study, work and invest in the UK'. This aims to control migration to limit non-EU economic migrants and minimize abuse of all migration routes. Alternatively, Australia has long had a strong pro-immigration policy to build its numbers and labour force. At the last census (2011), Australia had 21.5 million residents, over one-quarter of whom were born overseas, and nearly half of whom were either born overseas or had a parent who was.

As many governments in the advanced economies are aware, immigration can have a strong and long-lasting impact on population growth and structure. In general, migrants are young, increasing the percentage of the host country's working-age structure and the fertility rate of the population as a whole. Yet, while immigration will in the short term achieve immediate increases in TFRs, population growth, and labour market contribution, these are unlikely to achieve full replacement level. In addition, they are unlikely to be sustainable over the longer term, and indeed they may eventually contribute to a worsening of the demographic deficit, as the TFRs of the immigrant population falls and they themselves age. However, there are also considerable indirect effects of migration on promoting innovation, economic growth, and employment.

There is general agreement that migration will not prevent the ageing of populations or the demographic deficit, but it may slightly alleviate both.[11] By 2050, for example, at current childbearing rates, without immigration the European population will decline by some 40 million. It will take significant immigration of around 800,000 per year to maintain current population levels.[12] The number of migrants needed to maintain the working-age population, however, is highly contested. The International Organization for Migration (IOM), for example, has projected that if migration rates stay largely at their current levels, the working-age population in OECD countries will rise by 1.9 per cent between 2010 and 2020, a considerable fall compared to the 8.6 per cent growth seen between 2000 and 2010.[13] The IOM further predicts that while the incoming (aged 20–4) working-age cohorts in OECD countries were some 32 per cent larger on average than the outgoing retiring (aged 60–4) ones in 2005, for almost half the OECD countries the outgoing cohorts will be larger than the incoming ones, and by 2020 the incoming will be nearly 9 per cent smaller for the OECD as a whole. The United Nations further calculates that an average annual net migration of around 1.4 million people is required to keep the proportion of the working-age population in the European Union stable between 1995 and 2050,[14] and the World Bank forecasts that for Europe and Russia combined a migration of 3.3 million annually until 2025, and 4.1 million annually between 2025 and 2050,[15] is needed to maintain this status quo.

In terms of childbearing, first-generation immigrant women usually have higher levels of childbearing than host country women and thus immigration initially raises the TFR of the host country.[16] This arises for a variety of reasons: for example, the culture and values in the region of origin may encourage higher levels of childbearing. Some women migrate for marriage and family reunion,[17] while others will postpone childbearing in their home countries due to economic uncertainty or local conflict. Others may choose to wait until they have settled in a new country due to the disruption that moving with young children brings.[18] In addition, migrants may actually increase the childbearing rates of local women, for example because young male migrants may increase the pool of men available for marriage or partnerships, or female migrant carers may free local women from caring responsibilities for other family members—dependent older relatives or children—which then encourages them to have more children.[19]

The UK birth rate, for example, increased across the past decade through the large number of births to immigrants and to British women of minority ethnic status. The 2011 TFR of UK-born mothers is 1.84 and of non-UK-born mothers it is 2.21, resulting in a combined TFR of 1.93. Births to immigrant women currently account for around one-quarter of all live UK births, an increase from 16.4 per cent in 2001.[20] Immigrants are thus contributing substantially to the total number of UK births. There is, however, variation in migrant women's childbearing. For example, migrant women from Bangladesh, Morocco, Pakistan, and parts of sub-Saharan Africa typically have childbearing rates exceeding that of native populations in Europe, while those from Eastern Europe and the Caribbean have rates similar to Western European countries.[21]

However, while women born overseas may have higher TFRs, the childbearing rates of their daughters, the second generation of mothers, usually converge with the host country rate.[22] This seems to be due to the assimilation of the migrant populations into the host community,[23] non-assimilation but adoption of the socio-economic and cultural norms, and reducing childbearing in order to achieve higher social mobility.[24] In addition, it is likely that national welfare policies, employment patterns, and other institutional factors encourage migrants to reduce their childbearing.[25]

Immigration may also boost public finances. Several UK studies conclude that overall, migrants make a net contribution in the UK,[26] and Germany also sees a near 40 per cent decrease in the net tax burden through the admittance of immigrants.[27] In terms of taxation, for example, immigration increases the number of potential tax payers on whom future tax increases can be levied.[28] In addition, migrants are less likely than natives to use the provision of the welfare state.[29] In particular, given the young ages of most immigrants, there will be little demand on public sector finances, as they are likely to contribute taxes but leave before they pull down on old-age benefits such as pensions. For example, almost half of overseas-born immigrants to the UK emigrate again within five years, which, in addition, will lower the UK's old-age dependency ratio as they will not age in the UK.[30] Indeed, immigrants from Central and Eastern European countries make a positive contribution to the UK public finances as they are less likely than natives to live in social housing, they have a high labour force participation rate, they pay proportionately more than natives in indirect taxes, and they make much less use of benefits and public services.[31]

The final question is whether immigration improves the competitiveness and productivity of a host country. Evidence from the US suggests that migrants encourage new investment, improve efficiency, and increase innovation and entrepreneurship through increasing creativity.[32] Immigration also increases the size of the local economy, which can potentially lead to more competition and efficiency. International migration can indirectly affect regional competitiveness through the trade and international linkages, which result from a country's diasporas remaining in touch with their country and region of birth. Immigration may also have a positive effect on trade between the source country of the immigrants and the host country, as immigrants tend to have a preference for the products from their home countries, and furthermore can reduce transaction costs of bilateral trade with their home countries either through individual characteristics such as business contacts or through more generic traits such as language.[33]

Importance of human capital

It may be argued, however, that the most important policy that any government could introduce to ameliorate the negatives and promote the positives of age-structural change is to enhance the human capital of their population through education. We explored in some detail the importance of education in reducing child-bearing, as illustrated by Figure 43 which directly links contraceptive use to education. In addition, we now have evidence that not only does contraceptive use go up with female educational

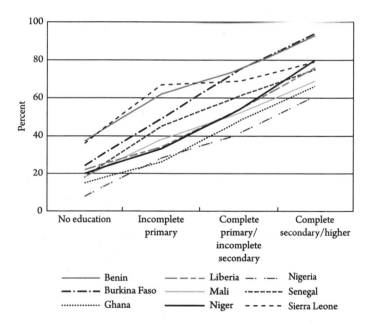

FIG 43 Ever-use of contraception by women's educational attainment, DHS data for nine countries in West Africa

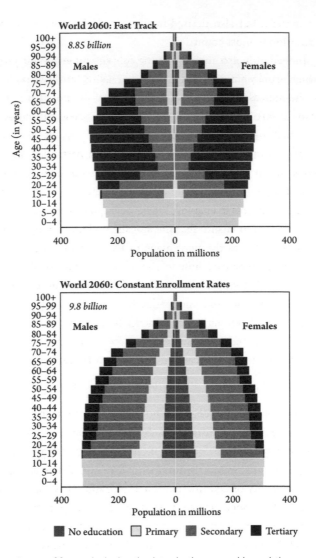

World 2060: Fast Track

8.85 billion

Males   Females

Age (in years)

400   200   0   200   400

Population in millions

World 2060: Constant Enrollment Rates

9.8 billion

Males   Females

400   200   0   200   400

Population in millions

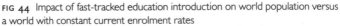

■ No education   □ Primary   ■ Secondary   ■ Tertiary

FIG 44 Impact of fast-tracked education introduction on world population versus a world with constant current enrolment rates

attainment, but also desired family size declines with increasing education in most countries.[34]

Indeed, it is also argued that the subsequent economic growth, which usually emerges after a period of falling fertility, may be due to the increased educational attainment of the population rather than the fertility transition itself.[35] While this view is disputed, it is clear that the demographic dividend is made possible with a more highly educated population (Figure 44). In particular, high skill levels within a population are increasingly required in the uptake and adoption of new technologies. And education not only plays an important role in enabling the demographic dividend, it also has the potential to ensure that the so-called window of opportunity does not close as the percentage of those of working age starts to decline. Enhanced human capital across the population and throughout individual lifespans through lifetime education enables a continuation of economic productivity, an important component of the second demographic dividend. It has also been argued that an increasingly educated society requires a lower childbearing rate to compensate for an increased percentage of older people.[36]

A confluence of twenty-first century challenges

Clearly, demographic change is not the only major global challenge of this century. A nexus of challenges have been identified. The Millennium Project, for example, identifies 15 global challenges (Figure 45). James Martin, founder of the Oxford Martin School at the University of Oxford, identified 17 (Table 8), while the Royal Geographical Society have 31 listed, including air pollution, urbanization, big data, food and water shortages, and natural disasters.

In this book, we have already brushed up against various major challenges for the twenty-first century—urbanization, terrorism, global health, the status of women, food, and water—illustrating

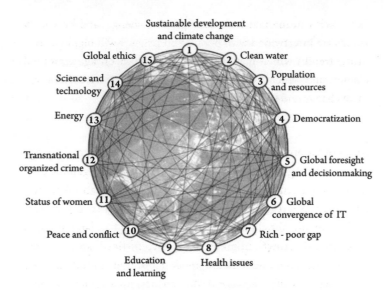

Sustainable development
and climate change

Global ethics (15)   (1)   (2) Clean water

Science and (14)   (3) Population
technology   and resources

Energy (13)   (4) Democratization

Transnational (12)   (5) Global foresight
organized crime   and decisionmaking

Status of women (11)   (6) Global
                        convergence of IT

Peace and conflict (10)   (7) Rich - poor gap

(9)   (8)

Education   Health issues
and learning

FIG 45 Fifteen global challenges from the Millennium project

(1) Climate change	(7) Protecting the biosphere	(13) Confronting existential risk
(2) Poverty	(8) Defusing terrorism	(14) Exploring transhumanism
(3) Steadying population growth	(9) Cultivating creativity	(15) Planning an advanced civilization based on leisure
(4) Achieving sustainable lifestyles	(10) Conquering disease	(16) Modelling the planet's systems
(5) Preventing all-out war	(11) Expanding human potential	(17) Bridging the skill and wisdom gap
(6) Dealing effectively with globalism	(12) The singularity	

TABLE 8 Seventeen great challenges of the twenty-first century

how each will interact with demographic change, and how such trends are intertwined with population issues. I will highlight two broad trends, which may have a major impact on age-structural change, and which I discuss in much more detail elsewhere: climate change and technological advances.[37]

The role of climate change

Many of the arguments we have made about age-structural change in the emerging economies and the potential for demographic dividends have been based on the concept that Asia, Latin America, and the MENA region will be the focus of twenty-first century economic growth. Yet climate shocks have already had large impacts on economic growth in many of these countries,[38] and it is recognized that an increase in the frequency and magnitude of such shocks will magnify the national consequences for economic growth. Indeed, it is being suggested that climate change may well impact upon sustainable economic development in a number of countries, causing significant problems in areas as diverse as health, water supply, agriculture, infrastructure damages, and financial and other economic services.[39]

As I have stated elsewhere,[40] seven of the cities recently identified as the top 50 in terms of their current and future importance to global business are at extreme risk from climate change-related extreme temperature and weather systems. Maplecroft's Climate Change Vulnerability Index (CCVI), which evaluates exposure to climate-related natural hazards and the sensitivity of populations, highlights the vulnerability of Dhaka, Bangladesh (1), Manila, the Philippines (2), Bangkok, Thailand (3), Yangon, Myanmar (4), Jakarta, Indonesia (5), Ho Chi Minh City, Vietnam (6), and Kolkata, India (7).

Coastal cities are particularly vulnerable as a sea-level rise of a few metres could result in widespread loss of coastal and deltaic areas.[41] For example, a sea-level rise of half a metre could result in 150 million people being threatened in some 136 port cities, with Kolkata, Mumbai, Dhaka, Guangzhou, Ho Chi Minh City, Shanghai, Bangkok, Rangoon, and Hai Phong being particularly vulnerable. Flooding, increased city temperatures, and cyclones could combine to impact upon the asset bases of many large cities—most in the emerging economies, such as Guangdong, Kolkata, Shanghai, Mumbai, Tianjin, Tokyo, Hong Kong, and Bangkok.[42] Significant risks to food and water security are predicted for South Asia, northern and sub-Saharan Africa, and parts of Russia.[43] Alternatively, many of the advanced economies, particularly in Northern and Western Europe, will provide environmentally sound locations in which to live and prove attractive to highly skilled migrants from environmentally challenged regions. Such negative aspects of climate change and their geographical focus on emerging economies and the least developed economies thus introduce an additional threat to the ability of such countries to capitalize on the potential bonus from age-structural change in these regions.

The impact of technological change

Technological change is advancing rapidly, and is having equally important interactions with demographic change, again particularly threatening the progress in emerging economies and the least developed economies:

> (We) are in the midst of a digital revolution that may be even more profound than the industrial revolutions of the past. Advances in robotics, cognitive computing and other digital technologies promise untold benefits in a world of leisure hard to imagine. But there is also a dark side to this technological change. It could lead to joblessness for most and extreme inequality, threatening economic health and political stability.[44]

Historically, new technology, such as nineteenth-century manu-facturing advances and twentieth-century computerization, sub-stituted for skilled labour through the replication and simplification of tasks. For example, the industrial revolution replaced a rela-tively small number of skilled artisans with large numbers of less-skilled factory workers.[45] However, the modern relationship between technological development and employment appears to be different, as advances in robotics and digital communications will principally reduce low-skilled and low-waged occupations, while highly skilled jobs requiring advanced cognitive and intui-tive skills will be protected[46] (though as we shall see this latter point is now contested). The twenty-first-century digital revolu-tion is thus displacing low- and middle-skilled jobs and providing job opportunities mainly for relatively skilled workers. Low-skilled workers across the globe will be affected by these trends, for example one estimation is that nearly half of all US jobs may be automatable over the next 20 years,[47] with transport, distribu-tion, and manufacturing being particularly affected. However, it is the emerging economies that are likely to be most vulnerable to job loss.

Asia, in particular, has benefited from the availability of cheap labour and the subsequent offshoring of jobs from Europe and the US. This promoted rural–urban migration as young people moved to the cities for manufacturing employment, which in turn drove national consumption, enabling the development of local markets and a thriving service economy. And as we saw in Chapter 4, this process is an essential part of the growing labour market required to turn the youth bulge into the demographic dividend. But things are already changing. With a steep rise in labour costs of up to 17 per cent a year, countries such as China are already pricing them-selves out of the cheap labour market. But rather than jobs moving to other Asian countries, such as Bangladesh and Vietnam, many are returning to the advanced economies, where they are being replaced by robotics. With a predicted 25 per cent increase in the use of robotics for manufacturing over the next ten years, advanced economies will increasingly replace their own manufacturing jobs and previously offshored jobs with automation. This has been illustrated by the US textile industry, which was decimated in the 1990s when the production process moved to China and India for mass cheap labour. However, the US industry is now being revitalized, as robotics and advanced digital machinery undertake the manufacturing of textiles with less than 10 per cent of the human workforce required, significantly reducing costs. And this is the second part of the technological story, as the majority of these new US textile jobs are for skilled technicians overseeing the robotics and automated work, with an increasing need for highly skilled workers in an increasingly automated world.

The intersection of age-structural change and the digital revolution has very clear implications for both emerging and advanced economies. Age-structural change in Asia, Latin America, and Africa is leading to a large youth bulge and labour supply at the very time when cheap labour employment in this part of the world is being threatened by automation. Over half of global robotic growth is occurring in China for example. Furthermore, not only is local automation occurring, but full-scale production is being withdrawn and returned to advanced economies as they are able to benefit from cheap manufacturing costs ensuing from automation. The jobs which will be available in both advanced and emerging economies will increasingly be for highly skilled technicians able to operate and work alongside robotics and other automated and digital systems, requiring greater investment in human capital and education—tasks which older workers with experience and training will be able to undertake in advanced economies. This thus reduces the need for skilled migrant labour from the South. And it is not only in manufacturing that such developments are being seen. Advanced voice recognition computers will have the ability to replace human labour in call centres; wordsmith programmes are already undertaking copy-editing and composing published news articles and business reports for agencies such as Associated Press. Again, advanced economies with an already highly educated and skilled workforce are moving to adapt to this, with the emergence of *mechatronics*, a combination of mechanical, electronic, and computer skills. It is thus argued that for human workers to compete successfully with robotics and computerization, they will have to acquire creative and social skills that enable them to undertake the sophisticated tasks currently beyond computerization. Here we have another challenge for emerging economies with their generally far less well-educated workforce.

I noted earlier that highly skilled jobs requiring advanced cognitive and intuitive skills will be protected in this revolution. Some, however, are questioning this, arguing that not only will white collar tasks such as article writing and data analysis be replaced by advances in machine learning, but advanced algorithms will threaten the majority of human tasks, including professional and creative work. IBM—which is at the forefront of advances in cognitive computing and machine learning—has created the Watson computer. This has the ability to scale—break down *expertise* into algorithms so that it can be learned by computers and widely disseminated—and is described as a machine 'that can really move into cognitive areas and start competing with people in terms of actual brain power',[48] a machine whose performance improves with feedback both from humans and the computer itself. Watson can also understand and process requests posed in everyday language.

However, the extent to which tasks requiring creative and social intelligence will be easily replicated by machines is debatable, and furthermore making predictions about technological progress is full of pitfalls, as witnessed by Minsky's infamous 1970 declaration that 'intelligent computers' would arrive during that decade. In addition, those parts of the world with strong regulations and political activism may slow down the incursion of technology into those professional and creative jobs and tasks that require human intuition and interpretation. This is not just about general resistance to the introduction of new technologies, which has historically been strong—for example, opposition to autonomous vehicles in some state of the US, such as California and Nevada, which are currently legislating for their use—or the public and medical resistance to the computerization of UK NHS medical records. Such opposition is usually eventually overridden. We are clearly moving on to a new page, where all human activity is under threat of computerization, automation, and transference into the digital and virtual space. In this new world, it may be argued that resistance will be at a different level and of a different type. This will be particularly and initially clear in the world of professional and creative jobs. Even if projects like IBM's Watson can successfully reproduce these tasks, people may choose to remain in control of these high-specification jobs. Economic employment is not just about money—it is about human contribution to the group of people they live within, and individual intellectual and creative satisfaction. It is thus not clear that current capitalist forces are sufficient to remove this from human activity. In those parts of the world with strong democratic political institutions, people may decide that the satisfaction achieved by undertaking collaborative contributory tasks overrides the economic consumption benefits which might occur with full computerization of all human activity. There may be evidence that computers can undertake creative and intuitive tasks 'better' than humans—but the resultant societal shifts might be seen as too great a sacrifice for this objective betterment.

Integrating demography into understanding

As we discussed in Chapter 4, varied regional and national economic growth has long been explained through political and governance structures. It is now clear that the demographic structure of the country also plays an important role. The varied separate regional development paths can be explained in part through the interaction of population growth and changing age structure with national economic, social, and political institutions. As Chapter 1 explored, economists typically believe that the demographic transition is something which follows on from economic growth. The advanced European and American economies experienced strong economic growth and the development of strong political structures in tandem with a long demographic age-structural transition. For some—economists in particular—this has become the accepted narrative. It is now clear that the narrative is a more complex process driven by socio-cultural as well as economic factors; that the implications for the demographic transition for the economy may be greater than economic factors for the transition; and that the transition has played as important a role in the process of human development. Indeed, the effect of changes in age structure on economic growth is now widely recognized in demography and population economics. An example of this is shown in Figure 46.

In particular, the emerging economies are facing a different relationship. East and South East Asia have had dramatic falls in fertility and mortality rates, leading to a shift in their age structures and vibrant economic growth but lower measures of political participation and democracy. While many countries in Latin America have

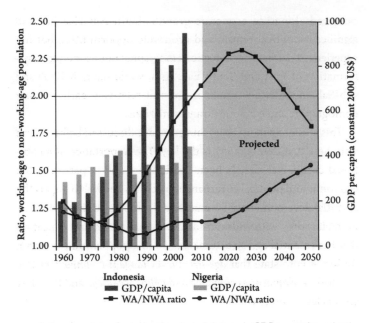

FIG 46 A comparison of actual and projected changes in GDP per capita and ratio of working-age (WA) to non-working-age (NWA) population for Indonesia and Nigeria reveal a close alignment

developed strong political institutions, it has, as a region, lagged behind in both economic growth and age-structural change. Similarly, the MENA region, while strong in some countries in terms of economic growth, is weak on political and demographic change. Finally, sub-Saharan Africa is currently weak in all three.

Overall, it can be seen that while economic and political structures are important, economic growth has only occurred without the prerequisite beneficial demographic change in exceptional circumstances. In Europe and Asia, with very different political institutions, age-structural change—in particular and crucially the percentage growth in workers and decline in younger dependents—

occurred alongside economic growth. Latin America has had significant political reform and economic opportunities, but has experienced neither the dramatic demographic nor economic transformation of East and South East Asia, while many MENA and sub-Saharan African countries are still relatively early in their demographic and economic transformations.

This is not to change everything we have discussed before—and state here that demography is the key. The importance of institutional change has already been emphasized, and in particular the economic and political governance structures needed to impart the essential development of human capital within a country. Furthermore, it is only with widespread advances in health and education that the essential age-structural change in a population can occur. Rather, it is to state that *age-structural change is as important to a country's development as economic and political change*, and that they are all clearly intertwined.

Twentieth-century institutions, twenty-first century challenges

The twenty-first century will face significant challenges from its changing demography—yet these will be tackled with inherited twentieth-century institutions.[49] We have noted education, health, and the ability of people to move in the light of population needs and pressures as being important to adapt to age-structural change. And yet all three face constraints inherited from the previous century.

While the flow of people, resources, and communications are increasingly cross-border, legal and political action is controlled in the main within national boundaries. There will be a quarter of a billion international migrants by 2030, crossing territories which still operate tightly regulated systems based on political states. There is little international flow of health, education, or welfare which transcends these national boundaries, but which is essential for both the well-being of the migrants, and for ensuring the best outcomes for them and their host and sending populations. Education is still instituted in old systems which emphasize foundation schooling to the neglect of advanced and lifetime learning and training. Yet as we saw, education is essential not only to reduce unwanted births, but also to prepare the largest cohort of young workers for the modern employment market, and to ensure that their skills and expertise are maintained across their ever-lengthening lifespans. Similarly, health systems are still predominantly focused on tackling acute diseases, in a world where chronic conditions and co-morbidities will be the largest health challenge.

As societies attempt to adjust successfully to age-structural change, a key question is thus how current national policies will influence the necessary societal adjustments and redistribution of resources to both maintain well-being across the life course, and within and between generations. For indeed, the major social goals held by most governments are achievable under all three demographic regimes we have described—whether a large percentage of young dependents, of young workers, or of older dependents.

Most governments wish to increase the general prosperity of their populations, reducing poverty and increasing both standards of living and health outcomes. Maximizing the benefits of both the first and second demographic dividends to provide resources for young and old dependents is important here. Many also recognize the goals of intragenerational and intergenerational fairness, which are used to frame policies related to redistributive transfer policies—either between differential income groups or generations. These may be used to mitigate the potential impact of public policy on the well-being of different birth cohorts to ensure that any effects arising from age-structural change are distributed fairly across older and younger cohorts in terms of facilitating health, education, employment, and access to societal resources. Successfully achieving these three broad goals should enable a fourth—that of promoting social cohesion.

Over the next 15 years some 2 billion new babies will be born, 2 billion children will need to commence school, and 1.2 billion young adults will need to find work. In addition, the fastest-growing age group globally will be the over 60s. Acknowledging the importance of age-structural change, and ensuring that it is integrated into national and international policymaking, will be essential as the globe transitions from a predominantly younger to a predominantly older world.

AFTERWORD

We started with the stories of three women, all in their 40s but living and experiencing very different lives. What of our future selves—the generations of tomorrow? Will their stories converge as the century progresses—or will we still see the inequalities of life opportunities for them as for their parents?

Three young girls describe their desired futures.

I would like many cows

Sola lives with her grandmother among the pastoralist Fulani tribe in Niger. The most important object in Fulani society is cattle. There are many names, traditions, and taboos concerning the traditional long-horned cattle, and the number of cows a person owns is a sign of their wealth. But cattle are not only prized possessions, they are a means of survival:

> My grandmother says I should go to school. But I don't want to go to school I want to stay home and help my grandmother. When I grow up I would like many cows. My husband will have many cattle, I will milk his cows and make the butter. I will walk with my friends to the market and sell the butter and cheese. If we have many cows and much butter to sell, I can have many daughters to help me, and sons to buy more cows. Then we will all go to market and make many beautiful clothes and blankets, like my grandmother does.[1]

I want to become a computer scientist

Fifteen-year-old Haitza Ortiz lives with her mother and younger sister in a poor suburb of Managua, Nicaragua's capital. Haitza's school starts in the afternoon, so she uses the morning to do chores around the house. She gets up at 5.30 a.m. every day to prepare breakfast for her sister and mother. Her sister Lupita goes to the same school, but in the morning, and her mother takes the bus to work as a maid at the other end of town. After Haitza's sister and mother leave the house, she feeds the animals and brings breakfast to an old man who lives next door. She then washes the dishes and the clothes. Afterwards, she begins to review her homework for school. A friend of Haitza's always comes by to study with her. After finishing her homework, Haitza cleans the house, then goes shopping and prepares lunch. The morning goes by fast and Haitza has to rush to take a bath before her friends arrive to accompany her on the 30-minute walk to school. Haitza studies at the San Luis School. She is in the second year of her secondary school. Haitza studies hard, with dreams of becoming a computer scientist, an ambition supported by her mother. 'My mother is always telling me I have to study to have a life better than hers. She had to drop out of school when she was 10 and was sent to work as a maid in the capital,' says Haitza.[2]

I want to be a fashion designer

Charlotte is 12 and lives with her parents in London—her mother is British, her father American. She is their only child. Charlotte travels by London Underground each day to her school some 15 minutes away:

Often I go with friends, sometimes alone, sometimes my Mum comes with me. I am very busy when I get home because I have to get my homework done and then I have extra classes or tennis or skating lessons. At the weekends, I usually have playdates or sleepovers with my friends. I go online in the evenings before bed to chat with my friends, because I do not wake up in time in the mornings! They are always a rush with Mum and Dad shouting at me to get out of bed as they have to go to work as well. When I grow up I will probably live with someone for a while and then we will have maybe one child—maybe two. After university, I want to go to fashion college and be a fashion designer. I also want to travel, maybe live in America for a while.[3]

APPENDICES

APPENDICES

APPENDIX I
Advanced economies: UN more developed regions

Albania	Estonia	Japan	Romania
Andorra	Faeroe Islands	Latvia	Russian Federation
Australia	Finland	Liechtenstein	Saint Pierre and Miquelon
Austria	France	Lithuania	San Marino
Belarus	Germany	Luxembourg	Serbia
Belgium	Gibraltar	Malta	Slovakia
Bermuda	Greece	Monaco	Slovenia
Bosnia and Herzegovina	Greenland	Montenegro	Spain
Bulgaria	Holy See	Netherlands	Sweden
Canada	Hungary	New Zealand	Switzerland
Channel Islands	Iceland	Norway	TFYR Macedonia
Croatia	Ireland	Poland	Ukraine
Czech Republic	Isle of Man	Portugal	United Kingdom
Denmark	Italy	Republic of Moldova	United States of America

Emerging economies: UN less developed regions, excluding least developed countries

Algeria	Cyprus	Libya	Saint Helena
American Samoa	Dem. People's Rep. of Korea	Malaysia	Saint Kitts and Nevis
Anguilla	Dominica	Maldives	Saint Lucia
Antigua and Barbuda	Dominican Republic	Marshall Islands	St Vincent and the Grenadines

Argentina	Ecuador	Martinique	Saudi Arabia
Armenia	Egypt	Mauritius	Seychelles
Aruba	El Salvador	Mayotte	Singapore
Azerbaijan	Falkland Islands (Malvinas)	Mexico	Sint Maarten (Dutch part)
Bahamas	Fiji	Micronesia (Fed. States of)	South Africa
Bahrain	French Guiana	Mongolia	Sri Lanka
Barbados	French Polynesia	Montserrat	State of Palestine
Belize	Gabon	Morocco	Suriname
Bolivia	Georgia	Namibia	Swaziland
Botswana	Ghana	Nauru	Syrian Arab Republic
Brazil	Grenada	New Caledonia	Tajikistan
British Virgin Islands	Guadeloupe	Nicaragua	Thailand
Brunei Darussalam	Guam	Nigeria	Tokelau
Cameroon	Guatemala	Niue	Tonga
Cape Verde	Guyana	Northern Mariana Islands	Trinidad and Tobago
Caribbean Netherlands	Honduras	Oman	Tunisia
Cayman Islands	India	Taiwan	Turkey
Chile	Indonesia	Pakistan	Turkmenistan
China	Iran (Islamic Republic of)	Palau	Turks and Caicos Islands
China, Hong Kong SAR	Iraq	Panama	United Arab Emirates
China, Macao SAR	Israel	Papua New Guinea	United States Virgin Islands
Colombia	Jamaica	Paraguay	Uruguay

Congo	Jordan	Peru	Uzbekistan
Cook Islands	Kazakhstan	Philippines	Venezuela
Costa Rica	Kenya	Puerto Rico	Vietnam
Côte d'Ivoire	Kuwait	Qatar	Wallis and Futuna Islands
Cuba	Kyrgyzstan	Republic of Korea	Western Sahara
Curaçao	Lebanon	Réunion	Zimbabwe

Least developed economies: UN least developed regions

Afghanistan	Equatorial Guinea	Mali	South Sudan
Angola	Eritrea	Mauritania	Sudan
Bangladesh	Ethiopia	Mozambique	Timor-Leste
Benin	Gambia	Myanmar	Togo
Bhutan	Guinea	Nepal	Tuvalu
Burkina Faso	Guinea-Bissau	Niger	Uganda
Burundi	Haiti	Rwanda	United Republic of Tanzania
Cambodia	Kiribati	Samoa	Vanuatu
Central African Republic	Lao People's Dem. Republic	Sao Tome and Principe	Yemen
Chad	Lesotho	Senegal	Zambia
Comoros	Liberia	Sierra Leone	
Dem. Rep. of the Congo	Madagascar	Solomon Islands	
Djibouti	Malawi	Somalia	

Data source: United Nations (2015) *World Population Prospects: The 2015 Revision*. Population Division of the Department of Economic and Social Affairs of the United Nations Secretariat, New York. Accessed 17 November 2015. With permission.

APPENDIX 2

Life expectancy at birth and life expectancy at age 60, 2010–15

Region or country	Life expectancy at birth		Life expectancy at age 60	
	Male	Female	Male	Female
World	68.28	72.74	18.71	21.54
More developed regions	75.09	81.47	20.79	24.61
Less developed regions	66.94	70.66	17.79	20.00
Least developed countries	60.73	63.59	16.67	17.84
Less developed regions, excluding least developed countries	68.31	72.15	17.91	20.23
Less developed regions, excluding China	65.05	69.07	17.42	19.64
Burundi	54.18	58.04	15.77	17.06
Comoros	61.20	64.50	15.32	17.02
Djibouti	60.04	63.24	16.85	18.08
Eritrea	60.90	65.18	13.67	16.94
Ethiopia	61.30	65.02	17.12	18.45
Kenya	59.08	62.17	17.06	18.44
Madagascar	63.02	66.00	16.21	17.48
Malawi	59.86	61.98	17.57	19.92
Mauritius	70.67	77.74	18.02	22.11
Mayotte	76.04	82.90	21.37	25.37
Mozambique	52.94	56.18	16.17	17.62
Réunion	76.04	82.90	21.37	25.37
Rwanda	59.65	66.30	17.12	18.45
Seychelles	68.69	77.91	16.88	21.92
Somalia	53.28	56.51	15.54	16.65
South Sudan	54.10	56.03	15.86	16.89
Uganda	55.67	58.83	16.62	17.92

United Republic of Tanzania	62.55	65.55	17.84	19.14
Zambia	57.16	60.33	16.99	18.36
Zimbabwe	53.60	55.95	16.80	18.18
Angola	50.20	53.17	15.09	16.27
Cameroon	53.74	56.02	15.84	17.01
Central African Republic	47.83	51.25	15.04	16.55
Chad	50.08	52.18	15.19	16.23
Congo	59.95	62.92	17.22	18.52
Democratic Republic of the Congo	56.67	59.53	16.05	17.14
Equatorial Guinea	55.87	58.57	16.26	17.45
Gabon	63.15	64.07	17.65	18.87
Sao Tome and Principe	64.23	68.19	17.49	18.84
Algeria	72.14	76.84	20.89	22.30
Egypt	68.71	73.05	16.05	18.39
Libya	68.79	74.41	16.84	19.64
Morocco	72.60	74.62	18.51	19.73
Sudan	61.60	64.60	17.17	18.32
Tunisia	72.30	77.04	17.74	21.22
Western Sahara	65.89	69.81	16.06	17.96
Botswana	61.80	66.51	15.92	18.13
Lesotho	49.19	49.59	14.49	16.22
Namibia	61.58	66.95	15.89	18.38
South Africa	54.85	59.11	13.47	18.06
Swaziland	49.69	48.54	15.30	17.20
Benin	57.77	60.61	14.96	16.12
Burkina Faso	56.73	59.33	14.68	15.44
Cape Verde	71.05	74.65	17.32	19.71
Côte d'Ivoire	50.21	51.85	13.83	14.40
Gambia	58.54	61.21	14.67	15.86
Ghana	60.06	61.97	15.03	16.01
Guinea	57.58	58.49	14.71	15.35
Guinea-Bissau	53.00	56.50	14.50	15.50
Liberia	59.29	61.21	14.84	15.82
Mali	57.44	56.98	15.14	15.30

(continued)

Region or country	Life expectancy at birth		Life expectancy at age 60	
	Male	Female	Male	Female
Mauritania	61.29	64.25	15.75	17.04
Niger	59.85	61.55	15.49	16.50
Nigeria	51.97	52.61	13.45	13.91
Senegal	63.86	67.61	15.71	17.43
Sierra Leone	49.65	50.74	12.97	13.05
Togo	58.28	59.68	14.65	15.42
China	73.97	77.02	18.32	20.60
China, Hong Kong SAR	80.91	86.58	23.45	28.16
China, Macao SAR	78.07	82.51	21.33	24.37
Dem. People's Republic of Korea	66.30	73.27	13.67	19.31
Japan	80.00	86.49	23.00	28.41
Mongolia	64.76	73.29	16.00	19.85
Republic of Korea	77.95	84.63	21.55	26.55
Other non-specified areas	76.43	82.30	21.67	24.92
Kazakhstan	64.29	73.87	14.38	19.18
Kyrgyzstan	66.35	74.29	15.50	19.60
Tajikistan	65.90	72.84	16.25	20.81
Turkmenistan	61.31	69.69	14.96	18.78
Uzbekistan	64.90	71.61	16.57	19.85
Afghanistan	58.67	61.06	14.95	16.47
Bangladesh	69.85	72.26	18.24	19.12
Bhutan	68.63	69.09	20.17	20.12
India	66.13	68.93	16.97	18.40
Iran (Islamic Republic of)	73.98	76.22	19.11	19.72
Maldives	75.40	77.41	18.96	20.06
Nepal	67.64	70.45	16.42	18.12
Pakistan	64.99	66.84	17.55	18.00
Sri Lanka	71.24	78.03	19.09	21.60
Brunei Darussalam	76.64	80.39	20.12	22.69
Cambodia	65.50	69.55	16.25	17.69
Indonesia	66.61	70.70	15.25	17.77
Lao People's Democratic Republic	64.14	66.84	15.75	17.40

Malaysia	72.21	76.88	18.43	20.13
Myanmar	63.58	67.66	15.67	17.55
Philippines	64.72	71.55	15.10	18.33
Singapore	79.59	85.61	22.47	27.47
Thailand	70.83	77.58	20.03	22.62
Timor-Leste	66.06	69.51	16.08	17.71
Vietnam	70.73	80.31	19.30	24.75
Armenia	70.74	78.39	17.04	21.95
Azerbaijan	67.54	73.77	16.43	19.89
Bahrain	75.58	77.42	18.92	20.02
Cyprus	77.69	82.17	20.44	23.77
Georgia	70.91	78.14	17.50	21.63
Iraq	66.99	71.44	16.21	18.64
Israel	80.18	83.82	23.23	25.71
Jordan	72.21	75.52	17.82	20.19
Kuwait	73.34	75.56	17.38	18.15
Lebanon	77.14	80.87	20.41	23.78
Oman	74.66	78.85	19.34	22.03
Qatar	77.10	79.68	20.51	21.93
Saudi Arabia	72.82	75.47	17.44	19.67
State of Palestine	70.74	74.66	17.22	19.72
Syrian Arab Republic	63.98	76.26	16.77	20.93
Turkey	71.53	78.12	18.63	22.71
United Arab Emirates	76.02	78.23	19.48	20.60
Yemen	62.18	64.88	15.41	17.11
Belarus	65.29	76.97	14.51	20.92
Bulgaria	70.64	77.56	17.00	21.17
Czech Republic	75.36	81.27	19.34	23.41
Hungary	71.23	78.54	17.53	22.06
Poland	73.06	81.14	18.75	23.86
Republic of Moldova	67.22	75.43	14.75	19.47
Romania	70.92	78.07	17.59	21.65
Russian Federation	64.15	75.55	15.19	20.66
Slovakia	72.24	79.73	17.71	22.42

(continued)

Region or country	Life expectancy at birth		Life expectancy at age 60	
	Male	Female	Male	Female
Ukraine	65.73	75.67	15.22	20.24
Channel Islands	78.45	82.39	21.34	24.90
Denmark	78.00	81.94	21.27	24.25
Estonia	71.57	81.05	17.87	23.87
Finland	77.60	83.40	21.62	25.61
Iceland	80.73	83.84	23.40	25.48
Ireland	78.40	82.74	21.72	24.93
Latvia	68.85	78.68	16.45	22.21
Lithuania	67.39	78.78	15.43	22.33
Norway	79.22	83.38	22.22	25.40
Sweden	80.10	83.71	22.82	25.58
United Kingdom	78.45	82.39	22.05	24.85
Albania	75.04	80.19	19.23	23.34
Bosnia and Herzegovina	73.71	78.82	18.46	21.77
Croatia	73.64	80.38	18.16	22.74
Greece	77.64	83.60	21.51	25.61
Italy	80.27	85.23	22.96	26.95
Malta	78.55	81.98	21.46	23.90
Montenegro	73.83	78.18	18.39	21.10
Portugal	77.43	83.50	21.53	25.62
Serbia	71.83	77.50	17.27	20.81
Slovenia	76.92	83.14	20.60	25.17
Spain	79.42	85.05	22.48	26.88
TFYR Macedonia	72.87	77.48	17.65	20.44
Austria	78.47	83.59	21.80	25.55
Belgium	77.95	83.02	21.66	25.44
France	78.76	84.87	22.88	27.24
Germany	78.18	83.06	21.59	25.23
Luxembourg	78.94	83.65	21.94	25.58
Netherlands	79.36	83.14	21.99	25.38
Switzerland	80.43	84.74	23.20	26.62
Antigua and Barbuda	73.29	78.21	19.95	22.78

Aruba	72.89	77.76	18.00	21.57
Bahamas	72.02	78.09	20.43	23.81
Barbados	72.91	77.71	17.76	21.15
Cuba	77.10	81.27	21.71	24.51
Curaçao	74.50	80.70	20.87	24.04
Dominican Republic	70.16	76.45	20.35	23.10
Grenada	70.78	75.59	17.53	19.89
Guadeloupe	76.83	83.98	22.20	26.57
Haiti	60.18	64.42	16.89	18.67
Jamaica	73.07	77.89	20.98	23.37
Martinique	77.79	84.36	22.40	26.84
Puerto Rico	75.19	83.17	21.06	25.90
Saint Lucia	72.17	77.57	19.22	22.90
Saint Vincent and the Grenadines	70.70	74.90	18.94	20.82
Trinidad and Tobago	66.87	73.84	16.10	20.24
United States Virgin Islands	77.24	82.92	20.43	25.88
Belize	67.19	72.72	15.75	18.39
Costa Rica	76.70	81.69	22.16	24.98
El Salvador	67.89	77.08	20.14	22.60
Guatemala	67.92	74.98	20.25	22.31
Honduras	70.39	75.40	20.70	23.41
Mexico	74.04	78.93	21.64	23.66
Nicaragua	71.38	77.48	21.02	23.40
Panama	74.34	80.49	22.51	25.29
Argentina	72.15	79.83	18.58	23.84
Bolivia (Plurinational State of)	65.34	70.21	20.02	22.17
Brazil	70.29	77.86	19.42	22.95
Chile	78.09	84.12	23.08	26.91
Colombia	70.19	77.39	20.08	22.53
Ecuador	72.82	78.37	21.75	23.93
French Guiana	75.75	82.58	19.52	25.04
Guyana	64.03	68.59	15.42	16.60
Paraguay	70.70	74.92	19.95	22.15
Peru	71.54	76.84	19.76	22.66

(continued)

Region or country	Life expectancy at birth		Life expectancy at age 60	
	Male	Female	Male	Female
Suriname	67.81	74.18	16.74	20.13
Uruguay	73.25	80.44	19.04	24.51
Venezuela (Bolivarian Republic of)	69.93	78.24	18.58	22.64
Canada	79.69	83.78	23.08	26.16
United States of America	76.47	81.25	21.76	24.72
Australia	79.93	84.28	23.28	26.45
New Zealand	79.71	83.35	23.17	25.79
Fiji	66.93	72.89	15.31	18.83
New Caledonia	73.55	79.31	18.32	22.65
Papua New Guinea	60.25	64.49	13.26	16.51
Solomon Islands	66.19	69.03	16.12	17.80
Vanuatu	69.59	73.60	16.89	19.22
Guam	76.14	81.47	19.77	24.21
Kiribati	62.55	68.93	15.52	17.78
Micronesia (Fed. States of)	67.99	69.85	16.50	17.97
French Polynesia	73.97	78.55	18.87	21.70
Samoa	70.02	76.39	16.41	21.44
Tonga	69.72	75.56	16.22	20.95

Data source: United Nations (2015) *World Population Prospects: The 2015 Revision.* Population Division of the Department of Economic and Social Affairs of the United Nations Secretariat, New York. Accessed 17 November 2015. With permission.

APPENDIX 3

Total Fertility, 2010–15 (children per woman)

Region or country	TFR
World	2.51
More developed regions	1.67
Less developed regions	2.65
Least developed countries	4.27
Less developed regions, excluding least developed countries	2.37
Less developed regions, excluding China	2.98
Burundi	6.08
Comoros	4.60
Djibouti	3.30
Eritrea	4.40
Ethiopia	4.59
Kenya	4.44
Madagascar	4.50
Malawi	5.25
Mauritius	1.50
Mayotte	4.10
Mozambique	5.45
Réunion	2.24
Rwanda	4.05
Seychelles	2.33
Somalia	6.61
South Sudan	5.15
Uganda	5.91
United Republic of Tanzania	5.24
Zambia	5.45
Zimbabwe	4.02

(continued)

Region or country	TFR
Angola	6.20
Cameroon	4.81
Central African Republic	4.41
Chad	6.31
Congo	4.95
Democratic Republic of the Congo	6.15
Equatorial Guinea	4.97
Gabon	4.00
Sao Tome and Principe	4.67
Algeria	2.93
Egypt	3.38
Libya	2.53
Morocco	2.56
Sudan	4.46
Tunisia	2.16
Western Sahara	2.20
Botswana	2.90
Lesotho	3.26
Namibia	3.60
South Africa	2.40
Swaziland	3.36
Benin	4.89
Burkina Faso	5.65
Cabo Verde	2.37
Côte d'Ivoire	5.10
Gambia	5.78
Ghana	4.25
Guinea	5.13
Guinea-Bissau	4.95
Liberia	4.83
Mali	6.35
Mauritania	4.69
Niger	7.63
Nigeria	5.74

Senegal	5.18
Sierra Leone	4.79
Togo	4.69
China	1.55
China, Hong Kong SAR	1.20
China, Macao SAR	1.19
Dem. People's Republic of Korea	2.00
Japan	1.40
Mongolia	2.68
Republic of Korea	1.26
Other non-specified areas	1.07
Kazakhstan	2.64
Kyrgyzstan	3.12
Tajikistan	3.55
Turkmenistan	2.34
Uzbekistan	2.48
Afghanistan	5.13
Bangladesh	2.23
Bhutan	2.10
India	2.48
Iran (Islamic Republic of)	1.75
Maldives	2.18
Nepal	2.32
Pakistan	3.72
Sri Lanka	2.11
Brunei Darussalam	1.90
Cambodia	2.70
Indonesia	2.50
Lao People's Democratic Republic	3.10
Malaysia	1.97
Myanmar	2.25
Philippines	3.04
Singapore	1.23
Thailand	1.53

(continued)

Region or country	TFR
Timor-Leste	5.91
Vietnam	1.96
Armenia	1.55
Azerbaijan	2.30
Bahrain	2.10
Cyprus	1.46
Georgia	1.81
Iraq	4.64
Israel	3.05
Jordan	3.51
Kuwait	2.15
Lebanon	1.72
Oman	2.88
Qatar	2.08
Saudi Arabia	2.85
State of Palestine	4.28
Syrian Arab Republic	3.03
Turkey	2.10
United Arab Emirates	1.82
Yemen	4.35
Belarus	1.58
Bulgaria	1.52
Czech Republic	1.45
Hungary	1.34
Poland	1.37
Republic of Moldova	1.27
Romania	1.48
Russian Federation	1.66
Slovakia	1.37
Ukraine	1.49
Channel Islands	1.46
Denmark	1.73
Estonia	1.59
Finland	1.75

Iceland	1.96
Ireland	2.01
Latvia	1.48
Lithuania	1.57
Norway	1.80
Sweden	1.92
United Kingdom	1.92
Albania	1.78
Bosnia and Herzegovina	1.28
Croatia	1.52
Greece	1.34
Italy	1.43
Malta	1.43
Montenegro	1.71
Portugal	1.28
Serbia	1.56
Slovenia	1.58
Spain	1.32
TFYR Macedonia	1.51
Austria	1.47
Belgium	1.82
France	2.00
Germany	1.39
Luxembourg	1.57
Netherlands	1.75
Switzerland	1.52
Antigua and Barbuda	2.10
Aruba	1.68
Bahamas	1.89
Barbados	1.79
Cuba	1.63
Curaçao	2.10
Dominican Republic	2.53
Grenada	2.18

(continued)

Region or country	TFR
Guadeloupe	2.17
Haiti	3.13
Jamaica	2.08
Martinique	1.95
Puerto Rico	1.64
Saint Lucia	1.92
Saint Vincent and the Grenadines	2.01
Trinidad and Tobago	1.80
United States Virgin Islands	2.30
Belize	2.64
Costa Rica	1.85
El Salvador	1.97
Guatemala	3.30
Honduras	2.47
Mexico	2.29
Nicaragua	2.32
Panama	2.48
Argentina	2.35
Bolivia (Plurinational State of)	3.04
Brazil	1.82
Chile	1.78
Colombia	1.93
Ecuador	2.59
French Guiana	3.48
Guyana	2.60
Paraguay	2.60
Peru	2.50
Suriname	2.40
Uruguay	2.04
Venezuela (Bolivarian Republic of)	2.40
Canada	1.61
United States of America	1.89
Australia	1.92
New Zealand	2.05

Fiji	2.61
New Caledonia	2.13
Papua New Guinea	3.84
Solomon Islands	4.06
Vanuatu	3.41
Guam	2.42
Kiribati	3.79
Micronesia (Fed. States of)	3.33
French Polynesia	2.07
Samoa	4.16
Tonga	3.79

Data source: United Nations (2015) *World Population Prospects: The 2015 Revision*. Population Division of the Department of Economic and Social Affairs of the United Nations Secretariat, New York. Accessed 17 November 2015. With permission.

NOTES AND REFERENCES

Chapter 1

1 The UN definitions are taken for the following three regions. Advanced economies: UN more developed regions; emerging Economies: UN less developed regions, excluding least developed countries; least developed economies: UN least developed regions. However, the definitions do have some incongruities, in particular the case of Japan which falls demographically into the advanced economy definition and will thus be included here.

2 All figures are based on current medium UN projections.

3 UN medium variant—United Nations, Department of Economic and Social Affairs, Population Division (2015): *World Population Prospects: The 2015 Revision.* New York.

4 Bongaarts, J. and Feeney, G. (1998) 'On the Quantum and Tempo of Fertility.' *Population Development Review* 24, 271–91; Bucht, B. (1996) 'Mortality Trends in Developing Countries: A Survey.' In Lutz, W. (ed.), *The Future Population of the World: What Can We Assume Today?* London: Earthscan, 133–48; Cliquet, R. L. (1991) 'The Second Demographic Transition: Fact or Fiction?' *Population Studies* 23. Strasbourg: Council of Europe; Lutz, W. and Goldstein, J. (2004) 'Introduction: How to Deal With Uncertainty in Population Forecasting?' *International Statistical Review* 72, 1–4; Van de Kaa, D. J. (1987) 'Europe's Second Demographic Transition.' *Population Bulletin* 42, 1–59; Vaupel, J. W. and Lundstrom, H. (1994) 'The Future of Mortality at Older Ages in Developed Countries.' In Lutz, W. (ed.), *The Future Population of the World: What Can We Assume Today?* London: Earthscan, 295–315.

5 In technical terms the TFR of a population is the average number of children that would be born alive to a woman during her lifetime if she

were to pass through and survive her childbearing years conforming to the age-specific fertility rates (ASFR) of a given year.

$$\text{TFR (per women)} = \frac{\text{sum of the single year ASFR}}{1000}$$

6 Harper, S. (2013) 'Population–Environment Interactions: European Migration, Population Composition and Climate Change.' *Environmental and Resource Economics*, 55(4), 525–41.

7 TFR for Niger = 7.63; life expectancy at birth = 60.7 years and life expectancy at age 60 = 16 years.

8 Average TFR for Malaysia = 1.97; life expectancy at birth = 75.3 years and life expectancy at age 60 = 19.7 years.

9 Average TFR for Italy = 1.43; life expectancy at birth = 82.8 years and life expectancy at age 60 = 25.1 years.

10 A vignette is a short piece of writing or acting that clearly shows what a particular person, situation, etc., is like.

11 The 'demographic dividend' is the rapid economic growth supported by changes in the age structure of a country's population as it transitions from high birth and death rates to low ones.

12 Lee, R. D. and Mason, A. (eds) (2011) *Population Aging and the Generational Economy: A Global Perspective*. Cheltenham: Edward Elgar.

13 Bloom, D. (2011) 'Population Dynamics in India and Implications for Economic Growth.' PGDA Working Paper No. 65.

14 Technically, here inequality is measured in terms of the Gini coefficient, which can be interpreted in terms of the expected difference in income between any two people chosen at random: the Gini coefficient is half the mean difference divided by the mean. See Atkinson, A. B. (2015) *Inequality: What Can Be Done?* Cambridge, MA: Harvard University Press.

15 Atkinson, A. B. (2015) *Inequality: What Can Be Done?* Cambridge, MA: Harvard University Press.

16 Von Weizsäcker, R. K. (1996) 'Distributive Implications of an Ageing Society.' *European Economic Review*, 40, 729–46.

17 Easterlin, R. A. (1987) 'Easterlin Hypothesis.' In J. Eatwell, M. Milgate, and P. Newman (eds), *The New Palgrave: A Dictionary of Economics*. New York: The Stockton Press, 1–4.

18 OECD (2008) *Growing Unequal? Income Distribution and Poverty in OECD Countries*. Paris: OECD publications.

19 Brandolini, A. and D'Alessio, D. (2001) 'Household Structure and Income Inequality.' Luxembourg Income Study Working Paper No. 254, Luxembourg.

20 UN medium variant, United Nations, Department of Economic and Social Affairs, Population Division (2015) *World Population Prospects: The 2015 Revision*. New York.

Chapter 2

1 The 1840s reports on the sanitary condition of the population in Cornwall and Devon ('Report on the Sanitary Condition of the Labouring Population and on the Means of Its Improvement.' London, May 1842) reveals that: 'open drains in some cases ran immediately before the doors of the houses, and some of the houses were surrounded by wide open drains, full of all the animal and vegetable refuse not only of the houses in that part, but of those in other parts of Tiverton. In many of the houses, persons were confined with fever and different diseases, and all I talked to either were ill or had been so: and the whole community presented a melancholy spectacle of disease and misery.' Similarly in Truro, where recently constructed sewers 'discharge themselves into the rivers...or after collecting filth from various localities, deposit a portion in catch pits here and there, and finally open on the surface, frequently in some street or lane, where a neglected deposit of a mixed animal and vegetable nature is allowed to become a probable source of annoyance or mischief.'

2 Szreter, S. (1988) 'The Importance of Social Intervention in Britain's Mortality Decline c. 1850? 1914: A Re-interpretation of the Role of Public Health.' *Social History of Medicine*, 1(1), 1–38.

3 Spini, G. and Casali, A. (1986) *Firenze*. Bari: Editori Laterza.

4 Sori, E. (1984) 'Malattia e demografia.' In F. Della Peruta (ed.), *Storia d'Italia—Annali, 7, Malattia e Medicina*. Torino: Einaudi, 541–73. C. Borro Saporiti (1984) 'L'endemia tubercolare nel secolo XIX: Ipotesi per ripensare un mito.' In F. Della Peruta (ed.), *Storia d'Italia—Annali, 7, Malattia e Medicina*. Torino: Einaudi, 844–75. E. Son (1984) 'Malattia

e demografia.' In F. Della Peruta (ed.), *Storia d'Italia—Annali, 7, Malattia e Medicina.* Torino: Einaudi, 541–73.

5 Sir John Simon, Medical Officer of Health for the city of London was appointed in 1848 to deal with the threat of cholera and other public health issues. 'Now here is a removable cause of death. These gases, which so many thousands of persons are daily inhaling,... rise from so many cesspools, and taint the atmosphere of so many houses, they form a climate the most congenial for the multiplication of epidemic disorders' (1848–9, 13). He was particularly concerned about London's water supply 'I consider the system of intermittent water supply to be radically bad... In inspecting the courts and alleys of the City, one constantly sees butts for the reception of water, either public, or in the open yards of the houses, or sometimes in the cellars; and these butts, dirty, mouldering, and coverless; receiving soot and all other impurities from the air; absorbing stench from the adjacent cesspool; inviting filth from insects, vermin, sparrows, cats, and children, their contents often augmented through a rain water pipe by the washings of the roof, and every hour becoming fustier and more offensive (1848–9, 23). Sir John Simon's Medical Officer of Health reports on the 'Sanitary Condition of London', 1848–55.

6 Castelli, L. (1893) *La poplazione e la mortalita del centennio 1791–1890. Edited by Ufizio di Igiene-Citta di Firenze.* Firenze: Stabilimento Tipografico Fiorentino.

7 Moggi-Cecchi, J., Pacciani, E., and Pinto-Cisternas, J. (1994) 'Enamel Hypoplasia and Age at Weaning in 19th-Century Florence, Italy.' *American Journal of Physical Anthropology*, 93(3), 299–306.

8 MacKeown, T. (1976) *The Modern Rise of Population.* London: Arnold.

9 Smith, F. B. (1979) *The People's Health 1830–1910.* London: Groom Helm Ltd.

10 Ferguson, P. P. (1998) 'A Cultural Field in the Making: Gastronomy in 19th-Century France 1.' *American Journal of Sociology*, 104(3), 597–641.

11 Knapp, V. J. (1997) 'The Democratization of Meat and Protein in Late 18th and 19th Century Europe.' *Journal of History*, 59, 541–51.

12 Knapp, V. J. (1997) 'The Democratization of Meat and Protein in Late 18th and 19th Century Europe.' *Journal of History*, 59, 541–51.

13 Goody, J. (1982) *Cooking, Cuisine and Class: A Comparative Sociology.* Cambridge: Cambridge University Press, 155.

14 Scharer, M. R. (1992) *Food History in Switzerland: A Survey of the Literature.* Leicester: Leicester University Press.

15 Fogel, R. (1986) 'Nutrition and the Decline in Mortality Since 1700: Some Preliminary Findings.' In S. Engerman and R. Gallman (eds), *Long-Term Factors in American Economic Growth,* 439–556.

16 Bengtsson, T. and Lundh, C. (1999) 'Child and Infant Mortality in the Nordic Countries Prior to 1900.' *Lund Papers in Economic History,* 66. Lund: Lund University.

17 McKeown, T., Record, R. G., and Turner, R. D. (1975) 'An Interpretation of the Decline of Mortality in England and Wales During the Twentieth Century.' *Population Studies,* 29(3), 391–422.

18 Fleming was awarded the 1945 Nobel Prize in Physiology and Medicine, along with Ernst Chain and Howard Florey, who helped develop penicillin into a widely available medical product.

19 Centers for Disease Control and Prevention (1999) 'Achievements in Public Health, 1900–1999: Changes in the Public Health System.' *Morbidity and Mortality Weekly Report,* 48(50), 1141–7.

20 Cooter, R. and J. Pickstone (2000) *Medicine in the Twentieth Century.* Amsterdam: Harwood Academic Publishers.

21 The theory of the epidemiological transition focuses on the complex change in the pattern of health and disease and the on the interactions between these patterns and their demographic, economic, and sociological determinants and consequences. See Omran, A. (2005) 'The Epidemiologic Transition: A Theory of the Epidemiology of Population Change.' *Millbank Q,* 83(4), 731–57.

22 Omran, A. (2005) 'The Epidemiologic Transition: A Theory of the Epidemiology of Population Change.' *Millbank Q,* 83(4), 731–57.

23 England, S., Loevinsohn, B., Melgaard, B., Kou, U., and Jha, P. (2001) 'The Evidence Base for Interventions to Reduce Mortality from Vaccine-Preventable Diseases in Low and Middle-Income Countries.' Commission on Macroeconomics and Health Working Paper No. WG5:10, World Health Organization.

24 WHO Global Program on Vaccines and Immunization (1996) *Progress of Vaccine Research and Development and Plan of Activities, 1996:*

Including Report of the Meeting of the Research and Development Technical Group (TRG), 10–11 June 1996. Geneva: WHO.

25 Leeson, G. W. (2014) 'Drivers of Demographic Change in Twentieth and Twenty-First Centuries.' In Harper, S. and Hamblin, K. (eds), *International Handbook on Ageing and Public Policy.* Cheltenham: Edward Elgar, 23–35.

26 Leeson, G. W. (2013) 'The Demographics of Ageing in Latin America, the Caribbean and the Iberian Peninsula, 1950–2050.' In Montes de Oca (ed.), *Envejecimiento—en America Latina y el Caribe.* Mexico: UNAM, 53–71.

27 While 40 was the average life expectancy for women in England at that time, for the few of Jane's class—lesser gentry—who had survived infancy, and not faced the perils of child bearing, the average expectancy was nearer to 50 years.

28 Cope, Z. (1964) 'Jane Austen's Last Illness.' *British Medical Journal,* 3, 182–83; Upfal, A. (2005) 'Jane Austen's Lifelong Health Problems and Final Illness: New Evidence Points to a Fatal Hodgkin's Disease and Excludes the Widely Accepted Addison's.' *Medical humanities,* 31(1), 3–11.

29 Wrigley, E. A., Davies, R. S., Oeppen, J. E., and Schofield R. S. (1997) *English Population History from Family Reconstitutions 1580–1837.* Cambridge: Cambridge University Press. Current Western figures are 10 per 100,000 births, though they still reach 10 per 1,000 in some parts of the least developed world.

30 Dribe, M. (2004) 'Long-Term Effects of Childbearing on Mortality: Evidence from Pre-Industrial Sweden.' *Population Studies,* 58(3), 297–310.

31 Biddiss, M. (2014) 'Jane Austen (1775–1817) and the Cultural History of Health.' *Journal of Medical Biography,* 22(3), 155–63.

32 Marshall, C. (1992) '"Dull Elves" and Feminists: A Summary of Feminist Criticism of Jane Austen.' *Persuasions,* 14, 39–45.

33 Biddiss, M. (2014) 'Jane Austen (1775–1817) and the Cultural History of Health.' *Journal of Medical Biography,* 22(3), 155–63.

34 It has been argued that fertility decline has never occurred in the absence of mortality decline, though there is some evidence that fertility decline did precede mortality decline in the US and France.

35 Fertility reduction is thus an equilibrating response to maintain population stability in the face of changing mortality regimes. Notestein,

F. W. (1945) 'Population: The Long View.' In Schultz, T. W. (ed.), *Food for the World*. Chicago: University of Chicago Press, 36–57. Easterlin, R. A. (1975) 'An Economic Framework for Fertility Analysis.' *Studies in Family Planning*, 6, 54–63. Easterlin, R. A. and Crimmins, E. M. (1985) *The Fertility Revolution: A Supply-Demand Analysis*. Chicago: University of Chicago Press.

36 Livi-Bacci, M. (1999) *The Population of Europe*. Oxford: Blackwell.

37 Zhao, Z. (1996) 'The Demographic Transition in Victorian England and Changes in English Kinship Networks.' *Continuity and Change*, 11(2), 243–72.

38 The Princeton European Fertility Project in the 1970s led to the development of the Princeton Indices, and concluded that European fertility decline was driven more by cultural diffusion around accepted family size and reproductive behaviour than by economic development.

39 Coale, A. J. and Watkins, S. C. (1986) *The Decline of Fertility in Europe: The Revised Proceedings of a Conference on the Princeton European Fertility Project*. Princeton, NJ: Princeton University Press.

40 Watkins, S. C. (1990) 'From Local to National Communities: The Transformation of Demographic Regimes in Western Europe, 1870–1960.' *Population and Development Review*, 241–72.

41 Lesthaeghe, R. (1983) 'A Century of Demographic and Cultural Change in Western Europe: An Exploration of Underlying Dimensions.' *Population and Development Review*, 9(3), 411–35.

42 Wilson, C. (1984) 'Natural Fertility in Pre-Industrial England, 1600–1799.' *Population Studies*, 38(2), 225–40.

43 Van Bavel, J. (2004) 'Deliberate Birth Spacing Before the Fertility Transition in Europe: Evidence from Nineteenth-Century Belgium.' *Population Studies*, 58(1), 95–107; David, P. A. and Mroz, T. A. (1989) 'Evidence of Fertility Regulation Among Rural French Villagers, 1749–1789.' *European Journal of Population*, 5(2), 173–206.

44 Herz, B. K. and Sperling, G. B. (2004) *What Works in Girls' Education: Evidence and Policies from the Developing World*. USA: Council on Foreign Relations Press; Shapiro, D. and Gebreselassie, T. (2009) 'Fertility Transition in Sub-Saharan Africa: Falling and Stalling.' *African Population Studies*, 23(1), 3–23; Klasen, S. (1999) 'Does Gender Inequality

Reduce Growth and Development? Evidence from Cross-Country Regressions.' World Bank Policy Research Report Working Paper No. 7. Washington, DC: The World Bank; Palloni, A., Novak, B., and D'Souza, R. L. (2012) 'Female Education, Low Fertility, and Economic Development.' Center for Demography and Ecology, University of Wisconsin-Madison Working Paper No. 2012–03. Madison, WI: University of Wisconsin-Madison.

45 Caldwell, J. C. (1980) 'Mass Education as a Determinant of the Timing of Fertility Decline.' *Population and Development Review*, 6(2), 225–55.

46 Bongaarts, J. (1997) 'The Role of Family Planning Programs in Contemporary Fertility Transitions.' In Jones, G. W., Douglas, R. M., Cladwell, J. C., and D'Souza, R. M. (eds), *The Continuing Demographic Transition*. Oxford: Clarendon Press, 422–43.

47 Davis, K., Bernstam, M. S., and Ricardo-Campbell, R. (1986) *Below-Replacement Fertility in Industrial Societies: Causes, Consequences, Policies*. Cambridge: Cambridge University Press.

48 Leeson, G. W. (2014) 'Drivers of Demographic Change in Twentieth and Twenty-First Centuries.' In S. Harper and K. Hamblin (eds), *International Handbook on Ageing and Public Policy*. Cheltenham: Edward Elgar, 23–35.

49 Leeson, G. W. (2014) 'Future Prospects for Longevity.' *Post Reproductive Health*, 20,(1), 11–15.

50 Leeson, G. W. (2014) 'Drivers of Demographic Change in Twentieth and Twenty-First Centuries.' In S. Harper and K. Hamblin (eds), *International Handbook on Ageing and Public Policy*. Cheltenham: Edward Elgar, 23–35.

51 Lutz, W., Sanderson, W., and Scherbov, S. (2001) 'The End of World Population Growth.' *Nature*, 412, 543–45.

52 Lutz, W., Skirbekk, V., and Testa, M. R. (2005) 'The Low-Fertility Trap Hypothesis: Forces that May Lead to Further Postponement and Fewer Births in Europe.' *Vienna Yearbook of Population Research*, 4, 167–92.

53 Blossfeld, H. P., Klijzing, E., Mills, M., and Kurz, K. (2006) *Globalization, Uncertainty and Youth in Society: The Losers in a Globalizing World*. New York/London: Routledge; Kreyenfeld, M. (2010) 'Uncertainties

in Female Employment Careers and the Postponement of Parenthood in Germany.' *European Sociological Review*, 26(3), 351–66; Sobotka, T., Skirbekk, V., and Philipov, D. (2011) 'Economic Recession and Fertility in the Developed World.' *Population and Development Review*, 37(2), 267–306.

54 Caldwell, J. C. (1980) 'Mass Education as a Determinant of the Timing of Fertility Decline.' *Population and Development Review*, 6(2), 225–55; Mills, M., Rindfuss, R. R., McDonald, P., and Te Velde, E. (2011) 'Why Do People Postpone Parenthood? Reasons and Social Policy Incentives.' *Human Reproduction Update*, 17(6), 848–60.

55 Morgan, S. P. and Rackin, H. (2010) 'The Correspondence Between Fertility Intentions and Behavior in the United States.' *Population and Development Review*, 36(1), 91–118; Iacovou, M. and Tavares, L. P. (2011) 'Yearning, Learning, and Conceding: Reasons Men and Women Change Their Childbearing Intentions.' *Population and Development Review*, 37(1), 89–123; Mills, M., Rindfuss, R. R., McDonald, P., and Te Velde, E. (2011) 'Why Do People Postpone Parenthood? Reasons and Social Policy Incentives.' *Human Reproduction Update*, 17(6), 848–60.

56 Lutz, W., Skirbekk, V., and Testa, M. R. (2005) 'The Low-Fertility Trap Hypothesis: Forces that May Lead to Further Postponement and Fewer Births in Europe.' *Vienna Yearbook of Population Research*, 4, 167–92; Lutz, W. and Skirbekk, V. (2005) 'Policies Addressing the Tempo Effect in Low-Fertility Countries.' *Population and Development Review*, 31(4), 699–720.

57 McDonald, P. (2008) 'Very Low Fertility: Consequences, Causes and Policy Approaches.' *The Japanese Journal of Population*, 6(1), 19–23.

58 Basten, S., Sobotka, T., and Zeman, K. (2013) 'Future Fertility in Low Fertility Countries.' Vienna Institute of Demography Working Paper No. 5/2013, Vienna.

59 Feng, W., Cai, Y., and Gu, B. (2013) 'Population, Policy, and Politics: How Will History Judge China's One-Child Policy?' *Population and Development Review*, 38, 115–29.

60 Le Li (2013) 'Despite Changes to One-Child Policy, Chinese Parents Say Having Two Kids is Too Expensive.' *NBC News*, 30 November. Available at <http://www.nbcnews.com/news/other/despite-changes-one-child-policy-chinese-parents-say-having-two-f2D11677167>.

61 Basten, S. and Gu, B. (2013) 'Childbearing Preferences, Reform of Family Planning Restrictions and the Low Fertility Trap in China.' Oxford Centre for Population Research Working Paper No. 61, Department of Social Policy and Intervention, University of Oxford; Basten, S., Lutz, W., and Scherbov, S. (2013) 'Very Long Range Global Population Scenarios to 2300 and the Implications of Sustained Low Fertility.' *Demographic Research*, 28, 1145–66; Zhenzhen, Z., Cai, Y., Feng, W., and Baochang, G. (2009) 'Below-Replacement Fertility and Childbearing Intention in Jiangsu Province, China.' *Asian Population Studies*, 5(3), 329–47.

62 Shapiro, D., Kreider, A., Varner, C., and Sinha, M. (2010) 'Stalling of Fertility Transitions and Socioeconomic Change in the Developing World: Evidence from the Demographic and Health Surveys.' Paper presented at the 36th Chaire Quetelet symposium in demography, Catholic University of Louvain, Belgium.

63 Bongaarts, J. (2008) 'Fertility Transitions in Developing Countries: Progress or Stagnation?' *Studies in Family Planning*, 39(2), 105–10; Ezeh, A. C., Mberu, B. U., and Emina, J. O. (2009) 'Stall in Fertility Decline in Eastern African Countries: Regional Analysis of Patterns, Determinants and Implications.' *Philosophical Transactions of the Royal Society B*, 364(1532), 2991–3007; Shapiro D. and Gebreselassie, T. (2008) 'Fertility Transition in Sub-Saharan Africa: Falling and Stalling.' *African Population Studies*, 23(1), 3–23; Bongaarts, J. (2006) 'The Causes of Stalling Fertility Transitions.' *Studies in Family Planning*, 37, 1–16.

64 Outside sub-Saharan Africa, stalling is now rare, with only one Asian/North African country and one Latin American country recently identified as stalling.

65 Machiyama, K. (2010) 'A Re-Examination of Recent Fertility Declines in Sub-Saharan Africa.' DHS Working Paper No. 68. Calverton (Maryland): ICF Macro.

66 Schoumaker, B. (2009) 'Stalls and Reversals in Fertility Transitions in Sub-Saharan Africa: Real or Spurious?' University of Louvain, Department of Population Science and Development, Working Paper No. 30, Belgium.

67 South Africa, Botswana, Namibia, Lesotho, and Swaziland. TFR from UN World Population Prospects, 2015 Revision.

68 Bongaarts, J. (2007) 'Fertility Transition in the Developing Countries: Progress or Stagnation?' *Studies in Family Planning*, 39, 105–10; Bongaarts, J. (2006) 'The Causes of Stalling Fertility Transitions.' *Studies in Family Planning*, 37(1), 1–16; Westoff, C. F. and Cross, A. R. (2006) 'The Stall in the Fertility Transition in Kenya.' *DHS Analytical Studies*, 9. Calverton, MD: ORC Macro.

69 See, for example, this leading article on fertility treatment: *The Economist* (2014) 'Fertility Treatment.' 8 March. Available at <http://www.economist.com/news/leaders/21598648-birth-rates-are-not-falling-africa-fast-they-did-asia-more-contraception-would>.

70 Howse, K. (2015) 'Fertility Stalling.' *Population Horizons*, 12(1), The Oxford Institute of Population Ageing.

71 Eastwood, R. and Lipton, M. (2011) 'Demographic Transition in Sub-Saharan Africa: How Big Will the Economic Dividend Be?' *Population Studies*, 65(1), 9–35.

72 Infant mortality rate (IMR): even in developed countries this is still a focus of concern, here deaths in the first year of life only exceeded by those over 40:

$$IMR = \frac{\text{deaths under 1 year of age}}{\text{total live births in a calender year}} \times 1,000$$

73 WHO (2014) 'Reaching Every Child: The Polio Programme Leaves Its Legacy.' Available at <http://www.who.int/features/2014/polio-programme/en/>.

74 WHO. Global Health Observatory Data Repository. Distribution of Causes of Death Among Children < 5 years (%). Available at <http://apps.who.int/gho/data/node.main.ChildMortREG100?lang=en>.

75 WHO (2002) *The World Health Report 2002—Reducing Risks, Promoting Healthy Life*. Geneva: World Health Organization.

76 UNICEF (2013) *Improving Child Nutrition: The Achievable Imperative for Global Progress*. New York: UNICEF.

77 Harper, C., Alder, H., and Pereznieto, P. (2012) 'Escaping Poverty Traps: Children and Chronic Poverty.' In Ortiz, I., Daniels, L. M., and Engilbertsdottir, S. (eds), *Child Poverty and Inequality New Perspectives*. New York: UNICEF.

78 OECD (2015) *Health at a Glance 2015: OECD Indicators*. Paris: OECD Publishing.

79 Centers for Disease Control and Prevention. National, Center for Health Statistics. Health Data Interactive <http://www.cdc.gov/nchs/hdi.htm> accessed 16 November 2015.

80 National Center for Health Statistics (US) (2015) *Health, United States, 2014: With Special Feature on Adults Aged 55–64*. Hyattsville (MD). Available at <http://www.ncbi.nlm.nih.gov/books/NBK299348/>.

81 The terms *cohort* and *generation* are often used loosely to mean the same concept. Technically, cohorts refer to a group who experienced an event at the same time: for example the 2000 birth cohort refers to those born in the year 2000; the 1990s birth cohort refers to those born in the last decade of the twentieth century. Each cohort has its own unique history. Cohort analysis charts the numbers and characteristics of cohorts over their lifetimes. It permits a comparison of attitudes and behaviours in relation both to different ages and different historical events. For example, for the cohort of women born in 1930 their 20s was a time of getting married and having children, defined by the socio-cultural norms of the 1950s; for the cohort of women born in 1970 their 20s was a time of singlehood and independence from new family ties defined by the socio-cultural norms of the 1990s. Generation is a more general term used in different contexts: those living together in an historical period—a generation of writers; those in the same birth cohort; vertical members of a family—grandfather, father, and child comprise three generations of the family; members of age groups in society; the gap between 'generations' in a family or society. Here I use cohort to mean a group who experienced an event at the same time, and generation to refer to family relations.

82 Leeson, G. W. (2011) 'Editorial: The Importance of Demography.' *Journal of Population Ageing*, 4(1), 1–4.

83 Vaupel, J. (2010) 'Biodemography of Human Ageing.' *Nature*, 464, 536–42.

84 Vaupel, J. (2010) 'Biodemography of Human Ageing.' *Nature*, 464, 536–42.

85 Olshansky, S. J. and Carnes, B. A. (2009) 'The Future of Human Longevity.' In Uhlenberg, P. (ed.), *International Handbook of Population Aging*. Netherlands: Springer, 731–45.

86 Haub, C. and Kaneda, T. (2014) *2014 World Population Datasheet.* Washington, DC: Population Reference Bureau. Available at <http://www.prb.org/publications/datasheets/2014/2014-world-population-data-sheet/data-sheet.aspx>.

87 Engelhardt, H. and Prskawetz. A. (2004) 'On the Changing Correlation Between Fertility and Female Employment Over Space and Time.' *European Journal of Population* 20(1), 35–62.

88 Beard, J. R., Officer, A. and Cassels, A. (2015) *World Report on Ageing and Health.* Geneva: World Health Organization.

89 Christensen, K., Doblhammer, G., Rau, R., and Vaupel, J. W. (2009) 'Ageing Populations: The Challenges Ahead.' *The Lancet,* 374(9696), 1196–208.

Chapter 3

1 Harper, S. (2013) 'The Golden Age: Ageing Populations and the Effect on National Economies.' Presentation to Henderson Global Investors, 16 July.

2 A retirement scheme where the plan beneficiaries decide how much they want to contribute either by having the specified amount regularly deducted from their pay check or by contributing the desired amount in a lump sum.

3 International Monetary Fund (2011) *The Challenge of Public Pension Reform in Advanced and Emerging Economies.* Washington, DC: IMF.

4 <http://www.worldbank.org/en/region/eca>.

5 <http://www.economist.com/sections/europe>.

6 Lee, R. and Mason, A. (2011) *Population Aging and The Generational Economy: A Global Perspective.* Cheltenham: Edward Elgar.

7 Ogawa, N., Matsukura, R., and Chawla, A. (2011) 'The Elderly as Latent Assets in Aging Japan.' In Lee, R. and Mason, A. (eds), *Population Aging and the Generational Economy: A Global Perspective.* Cheltenham: Edward Elgar, 475–87.

8 Three broad groupings are currently defined by the UN Population Division: youth dependents aged under 15; working age population aged 15–64; and elderly dependents aged 65 and over.

9 European Commission (2006) *The Demographic Future of Europe: From Challenge to Opportunity.* Brussels: European Commission Publications.

10 Eurostat. 'Projected Old-Age Dependency Ratios per 100 Persons, TSDDE511.' Publications of the European Communities. Accessed 16 November 2015.

11 This approach is related to the thinking around *structure* and *agency* and can be followed up in Giddens, A. (1979) 'Agency, Structure.' In *Central Problems in Social Theory: Action, Structure, and Contradiction in Social Analysis.* Berkeley: University of California Press, 49–95.

12 Gruber, J. and Wise, D. (1999) *Social Security and Retirement Around the World.* London: University of Chicago Press.

13 This is changing with the introduction in some states of moderate fees.

14 Börsch-Supan, A. and Wilke, C. B. (2004) 'The German Public Pension System: How it Was, How it Will Be.' National Bureau of Economic Research, Working Paper No. 10525, Cambridge, MA.

15 OECD (2010) 'Public and Private Pension Expenditure.' In *OECD Factbook 2010: Economic, Environmental and Social Statistics.* Paris: OECD Publishing.

16 Kluge, F. A. (2011) 'Labor Income and Consumption Profiles: The Case of Germany.' In Lee, R. and Mason, A. (eds), *Population Aging and the Generational Economy: A Global Perspective.* Cheltenham: Edward Elgar, 327–39.

17 National Transfer Accounts (NTAs) construct accounts by age and generation, including both public and private or familial transfers. NTA was launched as an international project in 2004 under the direction of Ronald Lee and Andrew Mason, with funding from the US National Institute of Aging of the National Institutes of Health. The NTA framework defines a transfer as a transaction that transfers a good, service, or cash from an individual belonging to one age group to an individual belonging to another age group with no expectation of compensation.

18 Social Security also includes survivor's benefits and disability insurance.

19 Neumark, D. (2009) 'The Age Discrimination in Employment Act and the Challenge of Population Aging.' *Research on Aging,* 31(1), 41–68.

20 Medicare, for the elderly and disabled, and Medicaid for the poor.

21 Bloom, D. E., Canning, D., and Fink, G. (2010) 'Implications of Population Ageing for Economic Growth.' *Oxford Review of Economic Policy,* 26(4), 583–612.

22 Lee, R. and Mason, A. (2006) 'Reform and Support Systems for the Elderly in Developing Countries: Capturing the Second Demographic Dividend.' *Genus*, 62(2), 11–35.

23 Lee, R. and Mason, A. (2006) 'What Is the Demographic Dividend?' *Finance and Development, IMF*, 43(3), 1–9.

24 OECD (2006) *Live Longer, Work Longer*. Paris: OECD.

25 Kulik, C. T., Ryan, S., Harper, S., and George. G. (2014) 'Aging Populations and Management.' *Academy of Management Journal*, 57(4), 929–35.

26 Institute of Medicine (US) Committee on the Long-Run Macroeconomic Effects of the Aging US Population (2012) *Aging and the Macroeconomy: Long-Term Implications of an Older Population*. Washington, DC: National Academies Press.

27 Jenkner, M. E. and Leive, A. (2010) 'Health Care Spending Issues in Advanced Economies.' Technical Notes and Manuals 10/16. Washington, DC: International Monetary Fund.

28 European Commission (2012) *The 2012 Ageing Report: Economic and Budgetary Projections for the 27 EU Member States (2010–2060)*. Brussels: European Commission.

29 Zweifel, P., Felder, S., and Werblow, A. (2004) 'Population Ageing and Health Care Expenditure: New Evidence on the "Red Herring".' *Geneva Papers on Risk and Insurance: Issues and Practice*, 29(4), 652–66. Available at <http://ssrn.com/abstract5605153>; Seshamani, M. and Gray, A. (2004) 'Time to Death and Health Expenditure: An Improved Model for the Impact of Demographic Change on Health Care Costs.' *Age and Ageing*, 33(6), 556–61.

30 Robine, J.-M. and Jagger, C. (2005) 'The Relationship Between Increasing Life Expectancy and Healthy Life Expectancy.' *Ageing Horizons*, 3, 14–21.

31 Zweifel, P., Felder, S., and Werblow, A. (2004) 'Population Ageing and Health Care Expenditure: New Evidence on the "Red Herring".' *Geneva Papers on Risk and Insurance, Issues and Practice*, 29(4), 652–66; Seshamani, M. and Gray, A. (2004) 'Ageing and Health Care Expenditure: The Red Herring Argument Revisited.' *Health Economics*, 13(4), 303–14.

32 Zweifel, P., Felder, S., and Meiers, M. (1999) 'Ageing of Population and Health Care Expenditure: A Red Herring?' *Health Economics*, 8(6), 485–96.

33 Nolte, E. and McKee, C. M. (2008) 'Measuring the Health of Nations: Updating an Earlier Analysis.' *Health Affairs*, 27(1), 58–71.

34 Stuckler, D. (2008) 'Population Causes and Consequences of Leading Chronic Diseases: A Comparative Analysis of Prevailing Explanations.' *The Milbank Quarterly*, 86(2), 273–326.

35 Howse, K. (2010) 'What Kinds of Policy Challenge Does Population Ageing Generate for Health Systems?' IARU Working Paper, Oxford.

36 Leeson, G. W. (2004) 'The Demographics and Economics of UK Health and Social Care for Older Adults.' Working Paper No. WP304, Oxford Institute of Population Ageing.

37 Seshamani, M. and Grey, M. (2002) 'The Impact of Ageing on Expenditures in the National Health Service.' *Age and Ageing*, 31, 287–94.

38 Breyer, F., Costa-Font, J., and Felder, S. (2010) 'Ageing, Health, and Health Care.' *Oxford Review of Economic Policy*, 26, 674–90; Zweifel, P., Steinmann, L., and Eugster, P. (2005) 'The Sisyphus Syndrome in Health Revisited.' *International Journal of Health Care Economics and Financing*, 5(2), 127–45.

39 Smith, S., Newhouse, J. P., and Freeland, M. S. (2009) 'Income, Insurance, and Technology: Why Does Health Spending Outpace Economic Growth?' *Health Affairs*, 28(5), 1276–84.

40 Fries, J. F. (1980) 'Aging, Natural Death, and the Compression of Morbidity.' *New England Journal of Medicine*, 303, 130–35; Fries, J. F. (1989) 'The Compression of Morbidity: Near or Far?' *The Milbank Quarterly*, 208–32.

41 Gruenberg, R. M. (1977) 'The Failure of Success.' *The Milbank Memorial Fund Quarterly*, 55, 3–24; Verbrugge, L. (1984) 'Longer Life but Worsening Health? Trends in Health and Mortality of Middle-Aged and Older Persons.' *The Milbank Memorial Fund Quarterly*, 62, 475–519; Olshansky, S. J., Rudberg, M. A., Carnes, B. A., Cassell, C. K., and Brody, J. A. (1991) 'Trading off Longer Life for Worsening Health: The Expansion of Morbidity Hypothesis.' *Journal of Aging and Health*, 3(2), 194–216.

42 Manton, K. G. (1982) 'Changing Concepts of Morbidity and Mortality in the Elderly Population.' *Millbank Quarterly*, 60, 183–244.

43 Manton, K. G. (2008) 'Recent Declines in Chronic Disability in the Elderly US Population: Risk Factors and Future Dynamics.' *Annual Review of Public Health*, 29, 91–113.

44 Yong, V. and Saito, Y. (2009) 'Trends in Healthy Life Expectancy in Japan: 1986–2004.' *Demographic Research*, 20, 467–94.

45 Yong, V., Saito, Y., and Chan, A. (2011) 'Gender Differences in Health and Health Expectancies of Older Adults in Singapore: An Examination of Diseases, Impairments, and Functional Disabilities.' *Journal of Cross-Cultural Gerontology*, 26(2), 189–203.

46 Unger, R. (2006) 'Trends in Active Life Expectancy in Germany Between 1984 and 2003: A Cohort Analysis with Different Health Indicators.' *Journal of Public Health*, 14(3), 155–63.

47 Modelling Ageing Populations to 2030 (MAP2030). Available at <http://www.newdynamics.group.shef.ac.uk/map2030-modelling-ageing-populations-to-2030.html>.

48 Gruber, J. and Wise, D. (1998) 'Social Security and Retirement: An International Comparison.' *American Economic Review*, 88(2), 158–63.

49 Kluge, F. A. (2011) 'Labor Income and Consumption Profiles: The Case of Germany.' In Lee, L. and Mason, A. (eds), *Population Aging and the Generational Economy: A Global Perspective.* Cheltenham: Edward Elgar 327–39.

50 Lee, R., Donehower, G., and Miller, T. (2011) 'The Changing Shape of the Economic Lifecycle in the United States, 1970 to 2003.' In Lee, R. and Mason, A. (eds), *Population Aging and the Generational Economy: A Global Perspective.* Cheltenham: Edward Elgar, 313–26.

51 Lee, R., Donehower, G., and Miller, T. (2011) 'The Changing Shape of the Economic Lifecycle in the United States, 1970 to 2003.' In Lee, R. and Mason, A. (eds), *Population Aging and the Generational Economy: A Global Perspective.* Cheltenham: Edward Elgar, 313–26.

52 Jagger, C., Matthews, R. J., and Comas Herrera, A. (2009). 'The Effect of Dementia Trends and treatments on Longevity and Disability Over the Next 20 Years.' XXXVI International Population Conference/ XXVI ème Congrès international de la population. Marrakech: IUSSP-UIESP.

Chapter 4

1 Republished with permission of *Foreign Affairs*, from Goldstone, J. (2010) 'The New Population Bomb.' *Foreign Affairs*, 89(1), 31–43; permission conveyed through Copyright Clearance Center, Inc.

2 LaGraffe, D. (2012) 'The Youth Bulge in Egypt: An Intersection of Demographics, Security, and the Arab Spring.' *Journal of Strategic Security*, 5(2), 65–80.

3 Daniel LaGraffe, Office of the Secretary of Defense, was on assignment to the Defense Plans Division of the Office of the Defense Advisor at the United States Mission to NATO. LaGraffe notes that the views expressed in this article are the author's and do not represent the views of the Department of Defense or the US government.

4 Minkov, A. (2009) 'The Impact of Demographics on Regime Stability and Security in the Middle East.' DRDC CORA-TM 2009–021; Technical Memorandum, Ottawa: Defence R&D Canada, Centre for Operational Research and Analysis.

5 Kenyon, P. (2009) 'Partnerships for Youth Employment. A Review of Selected Community Based Initiatives.' Employment Working Paper No. 33, International Labour Office, Youth Employment Programme.

6 Brainard, I., Chollet, D., and LaFleur, V. (2007) 'The Tangled Web: The Poverty-Insecurity Nexus.' In Brainard, L. and Chollet, D. (eds), *Too Poor for Peace? Global Poverty, Conflict, and Security in the 21st Century*. Washington, DC: The Brookings Institution, 1–30.

7 Macunovich, D. J. (2000) 'Relative Cohort Size: Source of a Unifying Theory of Global Fertility Transition.' *Population Development Review*, 26(2), 235–61.

8 Bloom, D. E. and Williamson, J. G. (1998) 'Demographic Transitions and Economic Miracles in Emerging Asia.' *The World Bank Economic Review*, 12(3), 419–55.

9 Collier, P. (2008) *The Bottom Billion: Why the Poorest Countries Are Failing and What Can Be Done About It*. New York: Oxford University Press.

10 Liotta, P. H. and Miskel, J. F. (2004) 'Redrawing the Map of the Future.' *World Policy Journal*, 21(1), 15–21; Cincotta, R. P., Engelman, R., and Anastasion, D. (2003) *The Security Demographic: Population and Civil Conflict after the Cold War*. Washington, DC: Population Action International.

11 Urdal, H. (2007) 'The Demographics of Political Violence: Youth Bulges, Insecurity, and Conflict.' In Brainard, L. and Chollet, D. (eds), *Too Poor for Peace? Global Poverty, Conflict, and Security in the 21st Century*. Washington, DC: The Brookings Institution, 90–100.

12 Kronfol, N. M. (2011) 'The Youth Bulge and the Changing Demographics in the MENA Region: Challenges and Opportunities.' The WDA-HSG Discussion Paper Series on Demographic Issues. WDA-Forum, University of St Gallen.

13 LaGraffe, F. (2012) 'The Youth Bulge in Egypt: An Intersection of Demographics, Security, and the Arab Spring.' *Journal of Strategic Security*, 5(2), 65–80.

14 Assaad, R. and Roudi-Fahimi, F. (2007) 'Youth in the Middle East and North Africa: Demographic Opportunity or Challenge?' Population Reference Bureau Policy Brief, Washington, DC.

15 Yousef, T. M. (2012) 'After the Spring: New Approaches to Youth Employment in the Arab World.' In World Economic Forum, *Addressing the 100 Million Youth Challenge Perspectives on Youth Employment in the Arab World in 2012.* Geneva: World Economic Forum.

16 World Economic Forum (2012) *Addressing the 100 Million Youth Challenge: Perspectives on Youth Employment in the Arab World in 2012.* Geneva: World Economic Forum.

17 Assaad, R. and Roudi-Fahimi, F. (2007) 'Youth in the Middle East and North Africa: Demographic Opportunity or Challenge?' Population Reference Bureau Policy Brief, Washington, DC.

18 Lam, D. (2014) 'Youth Bulges and Youth Unemployment.' *IZA World of Labor*, 26.

19 Minkov, A. (2009) 'The Impact of Demographics on Regime Stability and Security in the Middle East. DRDC CORA-TM 2009–021.' Technical Memorandum. Ottawa: Defence R&D Canada, Centre for Operational Research and Analysis.

20 Ahmed, M., Guillaume, D., and Furceri, D. (2012) 'Youth Unemployment in the MENA Region: Determinants and Challenge.' In World Economic Forum, *Addressing the 100 Million Youth Challenge: Perspectives on Youth Employment in the Arab World in 2012.* Geneva: World Economic Forum.

21 World Bank (2004) *Unlocking the Employment Potential in the Middle East and North Africa: Toward a New Social Contract.* Washington, DC: World Bank.

22 However, compared with other regions female labour participation is low: the private sector has not taken over from the public in employing

women, and this is compounded by the highly segregated labour markets along gender lines and private sector employers' unwillingness to take on the costs of maternity leave and child care. As a consequence only one-quarter of the region's women participate in the labour market, as opposed to around half globally.

23 Kuran, T. (2012) 'Building Arab Civil Society to Promote Economic Growth.' In World Economic Forum, *Addressing the 100 Million Youth Challenge Perspectives on Youth Employment in the Arab World in 2012.* Geneva: World Economic Forum.

24 Bloom, D. E., Canning, D., and Sevilla, J. (2003) *The Demographic Dividend: A New Perspective on the Economic Consequences of Population Change.* Santa Monica, CA: RAND.

25 Mohamad Al-Ississ (2012) 'The Access to Credit Dichotomy: Arab Financial Markets Caught Between the Pull of the Disenfranchised and the Push of the Entrenched.' In World Economic Forum, *Addressing the 100 Million Youth Challenge Perspectives on Youth Employment in the Arab World in 2012.* Geneva: World Economic Forum.

26 World Bank (2004) *Unlocking the Employment Potential in the Middle East and North Africa: Toward a New Social Contract.* Washington, DC: World Bank.

27 Mohamad Al-Ississ (2012) 'The Access to Credit Dichotomy: Arab Financial Markets Caught Between the Pull of the Disenfranchised and the Push of the Entrenched.' In World Economic Forum, *Addressing the 100 Million Youth Challenge Perspectives on Youth Employment in the Arab World in 2012.* Geneva: World Economic Forum.

28 Assaad, R. and Roudi-Fahimi, F. (2007) 'Youth in the Middle East and North Africa: Demographic Opportunity or Challenge?' Population Reference Bureau Policy Brief, Washington, DC.

29 Yousef, T. M. (2012) 'After the Spring: New Approaches to Youth Employment in the Arab World.' In World Economic Forum, *Addressing the 100 Million Youth Challenge Perspectives on Youth Employment in the Arab World in 2012.* Geneva: World Economic Forum.

30 Pitea, R. and Hussain, R. (2011) *Egypt after January 25: Survey of Youth Migration Intentions.* Cairo: International Organization for Migration; LaGraffe, D. (2012) 'The Youth Bulge in Egypt: An Intersection of Demographics, Security, and the Arab Spring.' *Journal of Strategic*

Security, 5(2), 65–80; Gilpin, R., Kandeel, A. A., and Sullivan, P. (2011) 'Diffusing Egypt's Demographic Time Bomb.' United States Institute of Peace Brief No. 81, Washington, DC.

31 LaGraffe, D. (2012) 'The Youth Bulge in Egypt: An Intersection of Demographics, Security, and the Arab Spring.' *Journal of Strategic Security*, 5(2), 65–80.

32 Postiglione, G. and Tang, J. T. H. (1997) *Hong Kong's Reunion with China: Global Dimensions*. Armonk, NY: M. E. Sharpe; Sweeting, A. (1995) 'Educational Policy in a Time of Transition: The Case of Hong Kong.' *Research Papers in Education*, 10(1), 101–29.

33 There is also a growing need to save to support those in retirement as life expectancy increases, which we consider in Chapter 6.

34 Bloom, D. E (2011) '7 Billion and Counting.' *Science*, 333, 562–9.

35 Chandrasekhar, C. P., Ghosh, J., and Roychowdhury, A. (2006) 'The "Demographic Dividend" and Young India's Economic Future.' *Economic and Political Weekly*, 5055–64.

36 UNESCO. Gross enrolment ratio, primary and secondary, female, 2010. Gross enrolment ratio by level of education. Accessed 16 November 2015.

37 Clifton, D. and Frost, A. (2011) *The World's Women and Girls 2011 Data Sheet*. Washington, DC: Population Reference Bureau.

38 World Bank (2015) *Adjusting to a Changing World*. East Asia and Pacific Economic Update, April 2015. Washington, DC: World Bank.

39 United Nations Population Fund (2011) *Impact of Demographic Change in Thailand*. Bangkok: UNFPA.

40 Leeson, G. W. (2011) 'Prepared or Not, Latin America Faces the Challenge of Aging.' *Current History, Journal of Contemporary World Affairs*, 110(733), 75–80.

41 Esteve, A., Garcia-Roman, J., Lesthaeghe, R., and Lopez-Gay, A. (2013) *The 'Second Demographic Transition' Features in Latin America: The 2010 Update*. Unpublished Manuscript. Barcelona: Centre d'Estudis Demogràfics.

42 Cleland, J., Bernstein, S., Ezeh, A., Faundes, A., Glasier, A., and Innis, J. (2006) 'Family Planning: The Unfinished Agenda.' *The Lancet*, 368(9549), 1810–27.

43 Bloom, D. E., Canning, D., Evans, D. K., Graham, B. S., Lynch, P., and Murphy, E. E. (2000) 'Population Change and Human Development in Latin America.' In Inter-American Development Bank, *Economic*

and *Social Progress in Latin America, 1999–2000 Report*. Washington, DC: IDB.

44 Bloom, D. E., Canning, D., Evans, D. K., Graham, B. S., Lynch, P., and Murphy, E. E. (2000) 'Population Change and Human Development in Latin America'. In Inter-American Development Bank, *Economic and Social Progress in Latin America, 1999–2000 Report*. Washington, DC: IDB.

45 Gribble, J. and Bremner, J. (2012) 'Achieving a Demographic Dividend.' *Population Reference Bureau*, 67(2).

46 United Nations Population Division, DESA (2015) *World Population Prospects: The 2015 Revision*. Accessed 27 November 2015.

47 Gribble, J. and Bremner, J. (2012) 'Achieving a Demographic Dividend.' *Population Bulletin*, 67(2).

48 Lee, R. and Mason, A. (2006) 'What Is the Demographic Dividend?' *Finance and Development, IMF*, 43(3).

49 India, Registrar General (2012) *Sample Registration System: Statistical Report 2010*. New Delhi: Vital Statistics Division, Office of the Registrar General as cited in Table 1, p. 164; Pradhan, I. and Sekher, T. V. (2014) 'Single-Child Families in India: Levels, Trends and Determinants.' *Asian Population Studies*, 10(2), 163–75.

Chapter 5

1 Roxburgh, C., Dörr, N., Leke, A., Tazi-Riffi, A., Van Wamelen, A., Lund, S., Chironga, M., Alatovik, T., Atkins, C., Terfous, N., and Zeino-Mahmalat, T. (2010) *Lions On the Move: The Progress and Potential of African Economies*. McKinsey Global Institute Report.

2 *The Economist* (2000) 'Hopeless Africa.' *The Economist*, 11 May. Available at <http://www.economist.com/node/333429>.

3 *The Economist* (2011) 'The Hopeful Continent: Africa Rising.' *The Economist*, 3 December. Available at <http://www.economist.com/node/21541015>.

4 Leke, A., Lund, S., Roxburgh, C., and Van Wamelen, A. (2010) 'What's Driving Africa's Growth?' *McKinsey Quarterly*, June.

5 Shimeles, A. (2014) 'Growth and Poverty in Africa: Shifting Fortunes and New Perspectives.' African Development Bank and IZA Discussion Paper No. 8751.

6 Sachs, J. and Warne, A. (1997) 'Sources of Slow Growth in African Economies.' *Journal of African Economies*, 6(3), 335–76.

7 Fosu, A. (2010) 'Does Inequality Constrain Poverty Reduction Programs? Evidence from Africa.' *Journal of Policy Modeling*, 32, 818–27.

8 Collier P., Elliott, V., Hegre, H., Hoeffler, A., Reynal-Querol, M., and Sambanis, N. (2003) *Breaking the Conflict Trap: Civil War and Development Policy*, Washington, DC: The World Bank and Oxford University Press.

9 Howse, K. (2014) 'Why Is Fertility Stalling and Why Does It Matter?' Population Horizons Working Paper No. 1, The Oxford Institute of Population Ageing.

10 Sachs, J. and Warne, A. (1997) 'Sources of Slow Growth in African Economies.' *Journal of African Economies*, 6(3), 335–76.

11 Radeny, M., Van Den Berg, M., and Schipper, B. (2012) 'Rural Poverty Dynamics in Kenya: Structural Declines and Stochastic Escapes.' *World Development*, 40(8), 1577–93.

12 Shimeles, A. (2014) 'Growth and Poverty in Africa: Shifting Fortunes and New Perspectives.' African Development Bank and IZA Discussion Paper No. 8751.

13 Ayogu, M. (2007) 'Infrastructure and Economic Development in Africa: A Review.' *Journal of African Economies*, 16 (Supplement 1), 75–126; Calderón, C., and Servén, L. (2010) 'Infrastructure and Economic Development in Sub-Saharan Africa.' *Journal of African Economies*, 19(AERC Supplement), i13–i87.

14 Cogneau, D. (2009) 'The Political Dimension of Inequality During Economic Development.' Document de Travail DT2009/10. Paris: DIAL.

15 Olowu, D. (2012) 'Gender Equality Under the Millennium Development Goals: What Options for Sub-Saharan Africa?' *Agenda: Empowering women for gender equity*, 26(1), 104–11.

16 These are Chad, Niger, Mali, Democratic Republic of Congo, Liberia, Central African Republic, and Sierra Leone. The UNDP's (2012) inequality measure is the Gender Inequality Index (GII), which reflects gender disadvantages in three dimensions: reproductive health, empowerment, and the labour market.

17 Field, E., Robles, O., and Torero, M. (2008) 'The Cognitive Link Between Geography and Development: Iodine Deficiency and

Schooling Attainment in Tanzania.' NBER Working Paper No. 13838, Cambridge, MA.

18 Blackden, C. M. and Wodon, Q. (2006) 'Gender, Time Use and Poverty in Sub-Saharan Africa.' World Bank Working Paper No. 73. Washington, DC: World Bank.

Blackden, C. M., Canagarajah, S., Klasen, S., and Lawson, D. (2006) 'Gender and Growth in Sub-Saharan Africa: Issues and Evidence.' UNU-WIDER Working Paper No. 2006/37, Helsinki.

19 Agénor, P. R., Canuto, O., and Da Silva, L. P. (2010) 'On Gender and Growth: The Role of Intergenerational Health Externalities and Women's Occupational Constraints.' World Bank Policy Research Working Paper No. 5492 Available at <http://ssrn.com/abstract= 1721330>.

20 Seguinoa, S. and Were, M. (2014) 'Gender, Development and Economic Growth in Sub-Saharan Africa.' *Journal of African Economies*, 23 (Supplement 1), i18–i61.

21 Howse, K. (2014) 'Why Is Fertility Stalling and Why Does It Matter?' Population Horizons Working Paper No.1, Oxford Institute of Population Ageing.

22 Garenne, M. (2008) *Fertility Changes in Sub-Saharan Africa*. DHS Comparative Reports No. 18. Calverton, MD: Macro International Inc.; Garenne, M. (2008) 'Situations of Fertility Stall in Sub-Saharan Africa.' *African Population Studies*, 23, 173–88; Garenne, M. L. (2011) 'Testing for Fertility Stalls in Demographic and Health Surveys.' *Population Health Metrics*, 9(59), 1–7.

23 Howse, K. (2014) 'Why Is Fertility Stalling and Why Does It Matter?' Population Horizons Working Paper No. 1, Oxford Institute of Population Ageing.

24 The alternative term *intermediate fertility variables* is also used

25 Howse, K. (2014) 'Why Is Fertility Stalling and Why Does It Matter?' Population Horizons Working Paper No. 1, Oxford Institute of Population Ageing.

26 Bongaarts, J., Franks, O., and Lesthaeghe R. (1984) 'The Proximate Determinants of Fertility in Sub–Saharan Africa.' *Population and Development Review*, 10(3), 511–37.

27 Moultrie, T. A. and Timæus, I. M. (2014) 'Rethinking African Fertility: The State In, and Of, the Future Sub-Saharan African Fertility Decline.' Annual Meeting of the Population Association of America, Boston, MA (Vol. 1).

28 Bongaarts, J. (2006) 'The Causes of Stalling Fertility Transitions.' *Studies in Family Planning*, 37(1), 1–16; Bongaarts, J. (2008) 'Fertility Transitions in Developing Countries: Progress or Stagnation?' *Studies in Family Planning*, 39(2), 105–10; Cetorelli, V. and Leone, T. (2012) 'Is Fertility Stalling in Jordan?' *Demographic Research*, 26(13) 293–318; Cleland, J., Bernstein, S., Ezeh, A., Faundes, A., Glasier, A., and Innis, J. (2006) 'Family Planning: The Unfinished Agenda.' *Lancet*, 368(9549) 1810–27; Ezeh, A. C., Mberu, B. U., and Emina, J. O. (2009) 'Stalls in Fertility Decline in Eastern African Countries: Regional Analysis of Patterns, Determinants and Implications.' *Philosophical Transactions of the Royal Society B: Biological Sciences*, 364(1532), 2991–3007.

29 Westoff, C. and Cross, A. (2006) *The Stall in the Fertility Transition in Kenya*. DHS Analytical Studies No. 9. Calverton, MD: ORC Macro.

30 Moultrie, T. A., Sayi, T. S., and Timæus, I. M. (2012) 'Birth Intervals, Postponement, and Fertility Decline in Africa: A New Type of Transition?' *Population Studies*, 66(3), 241–58.

31 Postponement of childbearing sees a lengthening between births; stopping is the cessation of childbearing; spacing is where the timing of childbearing is contingent on the age of the youngest child. Moultrie, T. A., Sayi, T. S., and Timæus, I. M. (2012) 'Birth Intervals, Postponement, and Fertility Decline in Africa: A New Type of Transition? *Population Studies* 66(3), 241–58.

32 Johnson-Hanks, J. (2004) 'Uncertainty and the Second Space: Modern Birth Timing and the Dilemma of Education.' *European Journal of Population*, 20(4), 351–73; Johnson-Hanks, J. (2007) 'Natural Intentions: Fertility Decline in the African Demographic and Health Surveys.' *American Journal of Sociology*, 112(4), 1008–43.

33 Moultrie, T. A., Sayi, T. S., and Timæus, I. M. (2012) 'Birth Intervals, Postponement, and Fertility Decline in Africa: A New Type of Transition?' *Population Studies*, 66(3), 241–58.

34 Chronic poverty is distinguishable by its duration and multidimensionality. Chronically poor people always or during a long period of their lives live below a poverty line.

35 Harper, C., Alder, H., and Pereznieto, P. (2011) 'Escaping Poverty Traps: Children and Chronic Poverty.' In Ortiz, I., Daniels, L. M., and Engilbertsdottir, S. (eds), *Child Poverty and Inequality New Perspectives*. New York: UNICEF.

36 Mensch, B. S., Bruce, J., and Greene, M. E. (1998) *The Uncharted Passage: Girls' Adolescence in the Developing World*. New York: Population Council.

37 Harper, C., Jones, N., and Watson, C. (2012) *Gender Justice for Adolescent Girls: Tackling Social Institutions. Towards a Conceptual Framework*. London: Overseas Development Institute.

38 Harper, C., Jones, N., and Watson, C. (2012) *Gender Justice for Adolescent Girls: Tackling Social Institutions. Towards a Conceptual Framework*. London: Overseas Development Institute.

39 Rowbottom, S. (2012) *Giving Girls Today & Tomorrow: Breaking the Cycle of Adolescent Pregnancy*. New York: UNFPA.

40 Harper, C., Jones, N., Presler-Marshall, E., and Walker, D. (2014) *Unhappily Ever After: Slow and Uneven Progress in the Fight against Early Marriage*. London: Overseas Development Institute.

41 Brown, G. (2012) *Out of Wedlock, Into School: Combating Child Marriage Through Education*. London: The Office of Gordon and Sarah Brown Limited; Malhotra, A., Warner, A., McGonagle, A., and Lee-Rife, S. (2011) *Solutions to End Child Marriage: What the Evidence Shows*. Washington, DC: ICRW; Nguyen, M. and Wodon, Q. (2012) *Global Trends in Child Marriage*. Washington, DC: World Bank.

Nguyen, M. C. and Wodon, Q. (2012) *Perceptions of Child Marriage as a Reason for Dropping Out of School: Results for Ghana and Nigeria*. Washington, DC: World Bank; UNFPA (2012) *Marrying Too Young: End Child Marriage*. New York: UNFPA; UNICEF Press Centre (2013) 'Child Marriages. 39,000 Every Day'. Joint news release from Every Woman Every Child/Girls Not Brides/PMNCH/United Nations Foundation/UNFPA/UNICEF/UN Women/WHO/World Vision/World YWCA, 13 March. Available at <http://www.unicef.org/media/

media_68114.html>; UNFPA (2012) *Marrying Too Young: End Child Marriage.* New York: UNFPA.

42 Jones, N., Presler-Marshall, E., Tefera, B., Emirie, G., Gebre, B., and Gezahegne, K. (2014) *Rethinking Girls on the Move: The Case of Ethiopian Adolescent Domestic Workers in the Middle East.* London: Overseas Development Institute.

43 Bantebya, G., Ochen, E., Pereznieto, P., and Walker, D. (2014) *Cross-Generational and Transactional Sexual Relations in Uganda: Income Poverty as a Risk Factor for Adolescents.* London: Overseas Development Institute.

44 Bantebya, G., Ochen, E., Pereznieto, P., and Walker, D. (2014) *Cross-Generational and Transactional Sexual Relations in Uganda: Income Poverty as a Risk Factor for Adolescents.* London: Overseas Development Institute.

45 Population Action International (2013) '10 Things You Should Know About Family Planning and Demographic Dividend.' Policy Brief. Washington, DC: Population Action International.

46 Population Action International (2013) '10 Things You Should Know About Family Planning and Demographic Dividend.' Policy Brief. Washington, DC: Population Action International.

47 Klasen, S. (1999) 'Does Gender Inequality Reduce Growth and Development: Evidence from Cross-Country Regressions.' Policy Research Report on Gender and Development Working Paper No. 7. Washington, DC: The World Bank.

48 Subbarao, K. and Raney, L. (1995) 'Social Gains from Female Education: A Cross-National Study.' *Economic Development and Cultural Change,* 44(1), 105–28.

49 Skirbekk, V. (2008) 'Fertility Trends by Social Status.' *Demographic Research,* 18(5), 145–80.

50 Rihani, M. A. (2006) *Keeping the Promise: Five Benefits of Girls' Secondary Education.* Washington, DC: Academy for Educational Development.

51 Harper, S. and Leeson, G. (2012) 'The Role of Education in Reducing Maximum World Population.' OIPA Working Paper. Oxford: Oxford Institute of Population Ageing.

52 Mlatsheni, C. and Leibbrandt, M. (2001) 'The Role of Education and Fertility in the Participation and Employment of African Women in

South Africa.' DPRU Working Paper No. 1/54. Cape Town: Development Policy Research Unit, University of Cape Town.

Palloni, A., Novak, B., and Rodrigues D'Souza, R. L. (2012) 'Female Education, Low Fertility, and Economic Development.' CDE Working Paper No. 2012–03. Madison, WI: Center for Demography and Ecology, University of Wisconsin-Madison.

53 Schultz, T. P. (1993) 'Investments in the Schooling and Health of Women and Men: Quantities and Returns.' *Journal of Human Resources*, 28(4), 694–734.

54 UNESCO (2012) *World Atlas of Gender Inequality in Education*. Paris: United Nations Educational, Scientific and Cultural Organization.

55 UIS (2011) *Financing Education in Sub-Saharan Africa: Meeting the Challenges of Expansion, Equity and Quality*. Montreal: Institute for Statistics, United Nations Educational, Scientific and Cultural Organization.

56 Madsen, L. (2013) 'Why Has the Demographic Transition Stalled in Sub-Saharan Africa?' *New Security Beat Blog*, Wilson Center, 7 August. Available at <http://www.newsecuritybeat.org/2013/08/demographic-transition-stalled-sub-saharan-africa/> accessed 28 September 2015.

57 Omilola, B. (2010) 'Patterns and Trends of Child and Maternal Nutrition Inequalities in Nigeria.' IFPRI Discussion Paper No. 00968, Figure 1. Washington, DC: International Food Policy Research Institute. Available at <http://ebrary.ifpri.org/cdm/ref/collection/p15738coll2/id/1578>.

58 Lee, R. and Mason, A. (2013) 'Population Change and Economic Growth in Africa.' Bulletin No 6. Honolulu, Hawai'i: National Transfer Accounts.

59 Mwabu, G., Muriithi, M. K., and Mutegi, R. G. (2011) 'National Transfer Accounts for Kenya: The Economic Lifecycle in 1994.' In Lee, R. and Mason, A. (eds), *Population Aging and the Generational Economy: A Global Perspective*. Cheltenham: Edward Elgar, 367–78.

60 Soyibo, A., Olaniyan, O., and Lawanson, A. O. (2011) 'The Structure of Generational Public Transfer Flows in Nigeria.' In Lee, R. and Mason, A. (eds), *Population Aging and the Generational Economy: A Global Perspective*', Cheltenham: Edward Elgar, 446–74.

Chapter 6

1 Harper, S. (2015) 'Waking Up to UK Futures.' Houses of Parliament Presentation, Parliamentary House of Science and Technology, June.

2 The United Nations, for example, defines population policies as actions taken explicitly or implicitly by public authorities in order to prevent, delay or address imbalances between demographic change and social, economic, and political goals.

3 Although recent research concludes that for most countries there are economic reasons why long-term fertility at levels somewhat below replacement would be preferable to replacement level. See Lee, R. and Mason, A. (2012) 'Is Fertility Too Low? Capital, Transfers and Consumption.' Presented at the Annual Meeting of the Population Association of America, San Francisco, CA.

4 OECD (2007) *Babies and Bosses: Reconciling Work and Family Life: A Synthesis of Findings for OECD Countries.* Paris: OECD.

5 D'Addio, A. C. and d'Ercole, M. M. (2005) 'Trends and Determinants of Fertility Rates: The Role of Policies.' OECD Social, Employment and Migration Working Paper No. 27. Paris: OECD; D'Addio, A. C. and d'Ercole, M. M. (2005) 'Policies, Institutions and Fertility Rates: A Panel Data Analysis for OECD Countries.' *OECD Journal: Economic Studies*, 41, June.

6 Davis, R. (2013) 'Promoting Fertility in the EU: Social Policy Options for Member States.' Library Briefing, Library of the European Parliament, 21 May.

7 Gustafsson, S. and Worku, S. (2005) 'Assortative Mating by Education and Postponement of Couple Formation and First Birth in Britain and Sweden.' *Review of Economics of the Household*, 3(1), 91–113.

8 Hoorens, S., Clift, J., Staetsky, L., Janta, B., Diepeveen, S., Jones, M. M., and Grant, J. (2011) 'Low Fertility in Europe: Is There Still Reason to Worry?' Monographs MG 1080. Cambridge: RAND.

9 Cleland, J., Bernstein, S., Ezeh, A., Faundes, A., Glasier, A., and Innis, J. (2006) 'Family Planning: The Unfinished Agenda.' *The Lancet*, 368(9549), 1810–27.

10 Sullivan, R. (2007) 'The Global, the Local, and Population Policy in Sub-Saharan Africa.' Institute for Research on Labor and Employment, University of California, Berkeley.

11 Coleman, D. A. (2002) 'Replacement Migration, or Why Everyone is Going to Have to Live in Korea: A Fable For Our Times from the United Nations.' *Philosophical Transactions of the Royal Society B: Biological Sciences*, 357(1420), 583–98; Espenshade, T. J., Bouvier, L. F., and Arthur, W. B. (1982) 'Immigration and the Stable Population Model.' *Demography* 19, 125–33; Espenshade, T. J. (2001) '"Replacement Migration" From the Perspective of Equilibrium Stationary Populations.' *Population and Environment*, 22, 383–400; Feld, S. (2000) 'Active Population Growth and Immigration Hypotheses in Western Europe.' *European Journal of Population*, 16, 3–39; Lesthaeghe, R. (2000) 'Europe's Demographic Issues: Fertility, Household Formation and Replacement Migration.' United Nations Expert Group Meeting on Policy Responses to Population Ageing and Population Decline. New York: United Nations Population Division; Pollard, J. H. (1973) *Mathematical Models for the Growth of Human Populations*. Cambridge: Cambridge University Press; Saczuk, K. (2003) 'Development and Critique of the Concept of Replacement Migration.' CEFMR Working Paper No. 4/2003. Warsaw: Central European Forum for Migration Research.

12 Lutz, W. and Scherbov, S. (2007) 'The Contribution of Migration to Europe's Demographic Future: Projections for the EU-25 to 2050.' Interim Report IR-07–024. International Institute for Applied Systems Analysis.

13 International Organization for Migration (2010) *World Migration Report 2010: The Future of Migration. Building Capacities for Change*. Geneva: International Organization for Migration.

14 UN (2000) *Replacement Migration: Is It a Solution to Declining and Ageing Populations?* New York: United Nations.

15 Holzmann, R. (2005) 'Demographic Alternatives for Aging Industrial Countries: Increased Total Fertility Rate, Labor Force Participation, or Immigration.' IZA Discussion Paper No. 1885. Bonn: Institute for the Study of Labor.

16 Andersson, G. (2004) 'Childbearing After Migration: Fertility Patterns of Foreign-Born Women in Sweden.' *International Migration Review*, 38, 747–5. Andersson, G. and Scott, K. (2005) 'Labour-Market Status and First-Time Parenthood: The Experience of Immigrant Women in Sweden, 1981–97.' *Population Studies*, 59, 21–38.

17 Booth, H. (2010) 'Ethnic Differentials in the Timing of Family Formation: A Case Study of the Complex Interaction Between Ethnicity, Socioeconomic Level, and Marriage Market Pressure.' *Demographic Research*, 23, 153–91; Milewski, N. (2007) 'First Child of Immigrant Workers and Their Descendants in West Germany: Interrelation of Events, Disruption, or Adaptation?' *Demographic Research*, 17, 859–96.

18 Milewski, N. (2007) 'First Child of Immigrant Workers and Their Descendants in West Germany: Interrelation of Events, Disruption, or Adaptation?' *Demographic Research*, 17, 859–96.

19 Roig Vila, M. and Castro Martín, T. (2007) 'Childbearing Patterns of Foreign Women in a New Immigration Country: The Case of Spain.' *Population*, 62(3), 351–80.

20 ONS (2014) *Childbearing of UK and Non-UK Born Women Living in the UK: 2011 Census Data*. London: Office for National Statistics.

21 Booth, H. (2010) 'Ethnic Differentials in the Timing of Family Formation: A Case Study of the Complex Interaction Between Ethnicity, Socioeconomic Level, and Marriage Market Pressure.' *Demographic Research*, 23, 153–91; Milewski, N. (2007) 'First Child of Immigrant Workers and Their Descendants in West Germany: Interrelation of Events, Disruption, or Adaptation?' *Demographic Research*, 17, 859–96; Sobotka, T. (2008) 'Overview Chapter 7: The Rising Importance of Migrants for Childbearing in Europe.' *Demographic Research*, 19(9), 225–48.

22 Kulu, H. (2005) 'Migration and Fertility: Competing Hypotheses Re-examined.' *European Journal of Population*, 21, 51–87; Toulemon, L. (2004) 'Fertility Among Immigrant Women: New Data, a New Approach.' *Population and Societies*, 400, 1–4; Genereux, A. (2007) 'A Review of Migration and Fertility Theory Through the Lens of African Immigrant Fertility in France.' MPIDR Working Paper WP 2007–2008. Rostock: Max Planck Institute for Demographic Research Sobotka, T. (2008) 'Overview Chapter 7: The Rising Importance of Migrants for Childbearing in Europe.' *Demographic Research*, 19(9), 225–48.

23 Coleman, D. (2006) 'Immigration and Ethnic Change in Low-Fertility Countries: A Third Demographic Transition.' *Population and Development Review*, 32(3), 401–46.

24 Forste, R. and Tienda, M. (1996) 'What's Behind Racial and Ethnic Fertility Differentials?' *Population and Development Review*, 22 (Supplement, *Fertility in the United States: New Patterns, New Theories*), 109–33.

25 Sobotka, T. (2008) 'Overview Chapter 7: The Rising Importance of Migrants for Childbearing in Europe.' *Demographic Research*, 19(9), 225–48.

26 Gott, C. and Johnson, K. (2002) 'The Migrant Population in the UK: Fiscal Effects.' Development and Statistics Directorate Occasional Paper No. 77. London: Home Office; Sriskandarajah, D., Cooley, L., and Reed, H. (2005) *Paying their Way: The Fiscal Contribution of Immigrants in the UK*. London: Institute for Public Policy Research.

27 Bonin, H., Raffelhüschen, B., and Walliser, J. (2000) 'Can Immigration Alleviate the Demographic Burden.' *FinanzArchiv*, 57, 1–21.

28 Brucker, H. (2002) 'Can International Migration Solve the Problems of European Labour Markets?' *Economic Survey of Europe*, 109–35.

29 Barrett, A. and McCarthy, Y. (2007) 'Immigrants in a Booming Economy: Analysing Their Earnings and Welfare Dependence.' *Labour*, 21(4–5), 789–808; Borjas, G. J. and Hilton, L. (1996) 'Immigration and the Welfare State: Immigrant Participation in Means-Tested Entitlement Programs.' *Quarterly Journal of Economics*, 111, 575–604; Brucker, H. (2002) 'Can International Migration Solve the Problems of European Labour Markets?' *Economic Survey of Europe*, 109–35. Bonin, H., Raffelhüschen, B., and Walliser, J. (2000) 'Can Immigration Alleviate the Demographic Burden.' *FinanzArchiv*, 57, 1–21.

30 Rendall, M. S. and Ball, D. J. (2004) 'Immigration, Emigration and the Ageing of the Overseas Born Population in the United Kingdom.' *Population Trends*, 116, 18–27.

31 Dustmann, C., Frattini, T., and Halls, C. (2010) 'Assessing the Fiscal Costs and Benefits of A8 Migration to the UK.' *Fiscal Studies*, 31, 1–41.

32 Audretsch, D. B.(2004) 'Sustaining Innovation and Growth: Public Policy Support for Entrepreneurship.' *Industry and Innovation*, 11(3), 167–91; Poot, J., Nana, G., and Philpott, B. (1988) *International Migration and the New Zealand Economy: A Long-Run Perspective*. Wellington: Institute of Policy Studies; Poot, J. (2008) 'Demographic Change and Regional Competitiveness: The Effects of Immigration and Ageing.' *International Journal of Foresight and Innovation Policy*, 4,

129–45; Quispe-Agnoli, M. and Zavodny, M. (2002) 'The Effect of Immigration on Output Mix, Capital, and Productivity.' *Economic Review—Federal Reserve Bank of Atlanta*, 87(1), 17–28; Saiz, A. (2003) 'The Impact of Immigration on American Cities: An Introduction to the Issues.' *Business Review*, Q4, 14–23; Audretsch, D. B. and Keilbach, M. (2004) 'Entrepreneurship Capital: Determinants and Impact.' Discussion Papers on Entrepreneurship, Growth and Public Policy No. 3704. Jena: Max Planck Institute for Research into Economic Systems.

33 Poot, J. (2008) 'Demographic Change and Regional Competitiveness: The Effects of Immigration and Ageing.' *International Journal of Foresight and Innovation Policy*, 4, 129–45.

34 Bongaarts, J. (2010) 'The Causes of Educational Differences in Fertility in Sub-Saharan Africa.' Working Paper No. 20. New York: Population Council.

35 Lutz, W. (2014) 'A Population Policy Rationale for the Twenty-First Century.' *Population and Development Review*, 40(3), 527–44.

36 Lutz, W. (2014) 'A Population Policy Rationale for the Twenty-First Century.' *Population and Development Review*, 40(3), 527–44.

37 Harper, S. (2016) *Population Environment and Technology*. Cambridge University Press.

38 International Monetary Fund (2003) *Fund Assistance for Countries Facing Exogenous Shocks*. Washington, DC: Policy Development and Review Department, International Monetary Fund.

39 IPCC (Intergovernmental Panel on Climate Change) (2007) *Climate Change 2007: The Physical Science Basis. Contribution of Working Group I to the Fourth Assessment Report of the IPCC*. Edited by S. Solomon, D. Qin, M. Manning, Z. Chen, M. Marquis, K. B. Averyt, M. Tignor, and H. L. Miller. Cambridge: Cambridge University Press; Shalizi, Z. and Lecocq, F. (2010) 'To Mitigate or to Adapt: Is That the Question? Observations on an Appropriate Response to the Climate Change Challenge to Development Strategies.' *The World Bank Research Observer*, 25(2), 295–321.

40 Harper, S. (2014) 'Demography and Environment'. In I. Goldin (ed.), *Is the Planet Full?* Oxford: Oxford University Press.

41 Huq, S., Kovats, S., Reid, H., and Satterthwaite, D. (2007) 'Editorial: Reducing Risks to Cities from Disasters and Climate Change.' *Environment and Urbanization*, 19(1), 3–15; Hare, W. L., Cramer, W., Schaeffer, M., Battaglini, A., and Jaeger, C. C. (2011) 'Climate Hotspots: Key Vulnerable Regions, Climate Change and Limits to Warming.' *Regional Environmental Change*, 11(1), 1–13.

42 Nicholls, R. J., Hanson, S., Herweijer, C., Patmore, N., Hallegatte, S., Corfee-Morlot, Château, J., and Muir-Wood, R. (2008) 'Ranking Port Cities with High Exposure and Vulnerability to Climate Extremes.' OECD Environment Working Paper No 1. Paris: OECD.

43 Risbey, J. S. (2011) 'Dangerous Climate Change and Water Resources in Australia.' *Regional Environmental Change*, 11(1), 197–203.

44 Abeshouse, B. (2015) 'The Tech Threat: Are Advances in Artificial Intelligence, Robotics and Other Technologies Leading to Fewer Jobs and More Inequality?' *Aljazeera*, 27 May. Available at <http://www.aljazeera.com/programmes/peopleandpower/2015/05/tech-threat-150527113050714.html>.

45 Frey, C. B. and Osborne, M. A. (2013) *The Future of Employment: How Susceptible are Jobs to Computerisation?* Oxford: Oxford Martin School.

46 Ford, M. (2015) *Rise of the Robots: Technology and the Threat of a Jobless Future*. New York: Basic Books.

47 Frey, C. B. and Osborne, M. A. (2013) *The Future of Employment: How Susceptible are Jobs to Computerisation?* Oxford: Oxford Martin School.

48 Watson Group Vice President, John Gordon, quoted in Abeshouse, B. (2015) 'The Tech Threat: Are Advances in Artificial Intelligence, Robotics and Other Technologies Leading to Fewer Jobs and More Inequality?' *Aljazeera*, 27 May. Available at <http://www.aljazeera.com/programmes/peopleandpower/2015/05/tech-threat-150527113050714.html>.

49 Harper, S. (2016) *Population Environment and Technology*. Cambridge University Press.

50 Cleland, J., Bernstein, S., Ezeh, A., Faundes, A., Glasier, A., and Innis, J. (2006) 'Family Planning: The Unfinished Agenda.' *The Lancet*, 368(9549), 1810–27.

51 United Nations, Department of Economic and Social Affairs, Population Division (2015) *World Population Prospects: The 2015 Revision*. Accessed 20 November 2015.

52 Bloom, D. E. (2011) '7 Billion and Counting.' *Science*, 333(6042), 562–69.

Afterword

1 Anonymized vignette.

2 UNICEF (2004) 'Real Lives: A Day in the Life of a Determined Schoolgirl.' Available at <http://www.unicef.org>.

3 Anonymized vignette from private communication.

INDEX